Advanced Praise for
THE WIN-WIN DIET

"Julie Wilcox's *The Win-Win Diet* makes me excited to pivot from my omnivore lifestyle to a flexitarian one. With her guidance in this book, I know that I'll be able to stick to my goals of becoming more plant-based without sacrificing joy."

—**Dana Cowin**, Founder, DBC Creative

"After working with Julie one-on-one, I hired her at TBWA\Chiat Day to set nutrition goals for my team and help achieve them. The guiding principles are now codified in her book, *The Win-Win Diet*. I'm so glad she's sharing her wisdom, recipes, and tips with the whole world so everyone can have the extraordinary opportunity we did to enhance health and well-being."

—**Nancy Reyes**, CEO TBWA\Chiat\Day NY

"As an Asian American, I was brought up with a high carb, sugar, and sodium diet and given junk food as an award. I also developed a late-night eating habit lifestyle. I wanted to change but as the saying goes, 'old habits die hard.' When I got to know Julie, I was inspired and decided to cut down on my meat consumption. After a few weeks and immediate changes in my physical and mental health, I decided to double down the success by becoming vegan. I have lost almost fifty pounds and have never had the energy and the strength that I have now. The win-win approach has not only helped me lose weight and see other physical changes but has also given me a new perspective on life."

—**Philip Chong**, President & CEO, Quincy Asian Resources Inc.

"Julie Wilcox is the real deal. Not only is she fiercely dedicated to her work, she walks her talk. Never have I met a woman so committed to leading a healthy lifestyle without falling prey to the dogma of fad diets we see today. We all have something to learn from her."

—**Jillian Turecki**, Relationship Expert

"Julie Wilcox takes you through all you need to know about healthy eating. *The Win-Win Diet* tells you how to live longer with enthusiasm and joy!"

—**Jana Klauer**, MD, author of *How the Rich Get Thin* and *The Park Avenue Nutritionist's Plan*

"The potential benefits of these health-promoting lifestyle recommendations are enormous, and readers will appreciate Julie Wilcox's patient, individualized, small changes approach to implementing and adhering to a more nutrition-conscious way of eating that can benefit not only each of us, but also reduces animal cruelty and improves planetary wellness—clearly a 'win-win' for all concerned."

—**Jonathan N. Tobin,** PhD, Professor, Department of Epidemiology & Population Health, Albert Einstein College of Medicine/Montefiore Medical Center

THE
WIN-WIN
DIET

THE WIN-WIN DIET

HOW TO BE PLANT-BASED
AND STILL EAT WHAT YOU LOVE

JULIE WILCOX

Post Hill PRESS

*To Mia, my inspiration in all things,
for whom I strive to set an example
of vibrant health and well-being.*

Contents

PART FIVE: SAMPLE MEAL PLANS   279

Introduction

The rise in popularity of plant-based eating spurs many questions: What exactly is a plant-based diet? Can I be plant-based and still eat some meat? If so, what kind and how much? How can I ensure that I will get all my nutrients when I am plant-based? How can I prevent myself from eating a meatless diet just as unhealthy as the one I ate before? Can being plant-based reverse my diabetes or hypertension, help me lose weight, or alleviate climate change? Can I afford to go plant-based? Will I be able to eat out? How will I be able to cook so many new foods? Are eggs good or bad? Is dairy inflammatory? And what is the truth about soy?

These are just some of the questions about this topical approach to eating I've been asked by clients, friends, and family, which is why I decided to write this book. I believe a plant-based diet is an excellent choice for most, because it offers many avenues and a large potential for personalization. What's more, becoming plant-based is easier than you think, as minimal changes yield a significant impact on your health, the environment, and animal welfare. In Part One of this book, I will explain the evidence in favor of a plant-based lifestyle, delve into the pros and cons of important foods to know about as you transition to this eating pattern, and lay out four approaches—flexitarian, pescatarian, vegetarian, and vegan—to help you determine where on the plant-based spectrum you fall. Then, in Part Two, I will help you put the principles from Part One into action, so that you can successfully maintain your plant-based lifestyle for life. In Part Three, I will show you how to transition from an omnivorous diet to the four I have selected, provide guides to help you assess yourself and your progress, and help you deal with different eating environments. I will explain why it is so important to find a community of support, be mindful, and self-nurture. Lastly, I will show you how to develop your own personalized diet with recipes in Part Four and sample meal plans in Part Five.

The buzz about plant-based diets is growing, and no matter what media you're into, it's hard to ignore. On Netflix, the documentaries *The Game*

Changers and *Forks Over Knives* profile people from all walks of life—from an average American struggling with various chronic metabolic diseases to an elite athlete—who have transformed their lives with plant-based diets. In a 2019 *New York Times* article, "The Meat-Lover's Guide to Eating Less Meat," Melissa Clark wrote about modifying her meat-heavy diet when she realized that cutting back on animal products, even a little, could benefit the environment. According to Clark, "The World Resource Institute, an environmental research group, recommends that wealthy nations cut their beef, lamb, and dairy consumption by forty percent to meet global emissions goals for 2050." Using the forty percent reduction amount as her guide, Clark decided to limit herself to two or three meals per week that included meat, seafood, or dairy. This plan has worked well for Clark and she's been able to stick with it for two reasons: she doesn't deprive herself of animal products completely, which she loves, and she is contributing to the wellness of the earth.

Clark is not alone. Bill Clinton, who remains devoted to a plant-based lifestyle, was one of the first to bring this style of eating to popular culture. In 2010, he announced he had become vegan to save his veins, arteries, and heart. In doing so, he also lost twenty-four pounds. Kim Kardashian has become an advocate of plant-based eating. Soccer star Alex Morgan swears by her plant-based diet as a performance-booster. In his acceptance speech for Best Actor at the 2020 Oscars, Joaquin Phoenix promoted plant-based eating by highlighting animal cruelty in food production. Even medical professionals, known to avoid giving nutrition advice for disease prevention and treatment, are increasingly endorsing plant-based eating, not only for their patients but also for themselves.

And the public is listening: according to surveys, polls, and industry sources, a significant percentage of American consumers over the age of eighteen are intending to eat less meat or cut it out of their diet all together (between 30 and 50 percent according to Rebecca Ramsing of the Johns Hopkins Center for a Livable Future, who conducted a survey on meat consumption habits from a representative sample of US households). Consumer-research powerhouse Gallup reported that plant-based food sales grew by 8.1 percent in 2017 and exceeded $3.1 billion in sales that same year. Global financial company UBS projects that the plant-based meat industry could grow from $4.6 billion, where it was in 2018, to $85 billion in sales in 2030, with annual increases of 28 percent.

Despite these facts, stats, and my personal adhesion to one type of plant-based diet (pescatarian), every individual is unique, so no single eating pattern fits all; what works for your sister, best friend, parents, or spouse may not be the right way to eat for you. But if you are thinking about becoming plant-based and want your new diet to last for the long term—whether your doctor suggested it for health reasons, you're interested in sustainability, a friend wants you to try it with them, or you just want to experience something different—this book will educate you about foods that can be a part of your shift and provide a guide to help you create an achievable, informed, and nutritious approach, uniquely tailored to your tastes, goals, and lifestyle. It's time to change your thinking from *losing*—weight, foods, satisfaction, and joy—to *winning*, on every front.

The win-win strategy operates on several levels. First, while implementing a framework that evidence shows has myriad health benefits, you will also be contributing to the well-being of the environment and animals. Second, despite what diet culture typically purports, you get to be plant-based without having to eliminate entire food groups or deprive yourself of foods you love. Third, with *The Win-Win Diet* you do not have to conform to an unattainable methodology made for the masses, but can design an entirely realizable, personalized plan, which has structure yet is flexible, balanced, and sustainable.

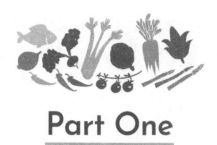

Part One

THE PLANT-BASED LIFE

What Is a Plant-Based Diet?

According to Oxford Languages, the definition of the term "plant-based" is "(of food or a diet) consisting largely or solely of vegetables, grains, pulses, or other foods derived from plants, rather than animal products." In conjunction with this meaning, "plant-based diet" is a catch-all term for any eating pattern mostly, but not wholly, comprised of vegetables, fruits, whole grains, legumes, nuts, seeds, and plant-based protein foods. Contrary to popular belief, therefore, this eating pattern can include modest amounts of animal-sourced foods such as eggs, dairy, fish, and yes, even meat. Plant-based diets also de-emphasize processed foods in favor of whole, natural foods. The expression "plant-based diet" can be misleading because most people associate the word "diet" with weight-loss strategy. While it is possible and common to lose weight by shifting to a plant-based eating pattern, the appeal is not just about getting slim. It's about developing a flexible, balanced, and sustainable eating pattern and lifestyle to address the increasing human health and environmental concerns related to food production and consumption, as well as animal welfare.

Interest among the general public in eating mostly or solely plant-based foods started to grow in the early 2000s, after author T. Colin Campbell and his son, Thomas M. Campbell II, published *The China Study* in 2006, which showed remarkable evidence that diets rich in animal products and processed, fast, and chemically derived foods drive disease and mortality, while whole, plant-based foods do the opposite. However, plant-based eating is hardly a modern fad. Vegetarianism dates back thousands of years to ancient Indian and Buddhist civilizations. During the life of Pythagoras, a meatless eating pattern was known as a "Pythagorean Diet." Throughout history, additional figures including Plato, Leonardo da Vinci, Descartes, Sir Francis Bacon, Voltaire, Rousseau, Einstein, George Bernard Shaw, and Gandhi promoted vegetarianism. Most early plant-based diet adopters grounded their rationale in compassion and nonviolence toward animals, religion, and perceived health benefits, which, with the advancements in nutrition science, we now know to be true.

The words we use to describe various approaches to plant-based eating, however, emerged much later. "Vegetarian," which refers to people who eat eggs and dairy but neither meat nor fish, appeared in the Merriam-Webster dictionary in 1839. "Vegan," defined as vegetarians who exclude all animal-based products, appeared in 1944. It wasn't until 1993 that "pescatarian" emerged as a term for those who eat fish, eggs, and dairy, but not meat (*pesce* is the Italian word for fish) and, more recently, "flexitarian" entered the lexicon, to describe a person who eats mostly vegetarian food, but also small amounts of meat and fish. The Mediterranean diet, DASH diet, VB6, fruitarian diet, reducetarian diet, and still others, qualify as plant-based too. The evidence-based reasons I chose the flexitarian, pescatarian, vegetarian, and vegan diets on which to focus are: 1) They follow a continuum, from limited meat consumption to consumption that is completely animal product-free, and thus appeal to many people with different tastes, preferences, and needs. 2) They are balanced and in line with public health objectives and evidence on healthy eating. 3) They can vastly improve health and reduce mortality. 4) They significantly reduce harm to the environment and animals. If you are still confused about what you can and can't eat on a plant-based diet, don't worry—that's what this book is for. But for now, perhaps the most straightforward way to think about what "plant-based" means is Michael Pollan's famous seven-word guide: "Eat food. Not too much. Mostly plants."

Why Now?

There are four major answers to the question of why plant-based diets are exploding in popularity today: the global prevalence of chronic disease due to the overly processed salt-, sugar-, and fat-rich Western diet, which has encroached on the rest of the world; the evolution of nutrition science, which has unveiled new research supporting the health benefits of plant-based living; climate change and expanding interest in sustainability; and the mindfulness movement, which has renewed people's concerns over animal welfare. The novel coronavirus, which evidence indicates is exacerbated by some health conditions caused by poor diet choices, is yet another emerging reason. Let's take a brief look at each of the four larger issues.

The Current State of Our Diets

Poor diet, chronic disease, and premature mortality are no longer solely America's problem. Obesity, type 2 diabetes, and cardiovascular disease (CVD)—all diet-related illnesses—are prevalent globally. Worldwide, obesity rates have tripled since 1975, due to calorie-dense, nutrient-imbalanced diets. In 2016, 13 percent of the global adult population was obese and 39 percent overweight, amounting to two billion people total. In the US alone, between 2015 and 2016, 39 percent of adults over the age of twenty were obese and 71.6 percent overweight. The age-adjusted prevalence among adults with obesity in the US from 2017 to 2018 rose to just over 42 percent. Both "obese" (defined as a BMI greater than 30) and "overweight" (defined as a BMI greater than 25) are major risk factors for cardiovascular disease, cancer, type 2 diabetes, and now COVID-19. According to the World Health Organization, cardiovascular disease ranks as the leading cause of mortality worldwide and is responsible for 31 percent or 17.9 million deaths each year. Cancer is the second leading cause of death in the world and accounts for approximately 16.5 percent or 9.6 million deaths. Diabetes, which more than doubled in prevalence between 1980 and 2014, is now ranked as the seventh leading cause of death, accounting for 8.5 percent or 1.6 million deaths globally. According to the CDC, 48 percent of hospitalized patients with COVID-19 are obese.

Decades of scientific research show that the biggest risk factors for these diseases are low consumption of fruits, vegetables, and whole grains, and high intake of meat and processed food, a style of eating that has spread from high-income countries to the developing world. As countries with emerging-market economies have become wealthier and more urbanized, the invasion of low-cost, low-quality convenience foods has increased consumption of meat to amounts that exceed healthy levels. (In the United States, meat consumption already exceeds recommendations from the 2015–2020 USDA guidelines by 20 to 60 percent.) Simultaneously, chronic disease and mortality have increased. If the world continues on this path—with global population expected to reach 9.8 billion in 2050 (up from seven billion in 2010), overall food demand projected to increase by 50 percent, and demand for animal-sourced foods forecasted to grow by 70 percent—the chances of achieving a sustainable food future are grim. A plant-based life is the preeminent means by which we can stymie and reverse these ominous health trends.

Health Benefits

Several years ago, I had a client seeking to manage her symptoms of polycystic ovary syndrome (PCOS). Like many women with this condition (one in ten women of childbearing age have it), she suffered from persistent abdominal pain, irregular periods, and infertility. During our initial assessment, I learned she was an omnivore. She ate meat once a day, loved dairy and eggs, and had a weakness for Doritos. Given this information, I asked her to try a plant-based diet, which studies have shown can significantly improve symptoms of PCOS and even help women who have not been able to conceive have babies. Over the course of six months, my client gradually eliminated red meat from her diet (she still ate white meat a couple of times a month), reduced her egg and dairy consumption, and stopped eating processed foods all together. The result? Her abdominal pain subsided, her periods became more regular, she lost weight, and, lo and behold, she got pregnant!

Health benefits are usually at the top of the list for people who want to learn more about plant-based diets. Frequently, interest is sparked after a doctor's visit. Perhaps your physician informs you that you need to reduce your blood pressure, cholesterol, weight, or blood glucose—factors that put you at risk for cardiac events, metabolic disorders, and other diseases. Possibly you complain of wanting to feel more energized, focused, and clear-minded, or you want to sleep more deeply. Maybe you learn you are leptin-resistant and never feel satiated after a meal, or that your ghrelin is on overdrive, making you feel hungry all the time. (Leptin is the hormone that signals the brain we are full and ghrelin that we are hungry.)

And the health objectives for going plant-based don't have to stem from a negative place. Athletes who want to improve their performance go plant-based. People who want to instill healthy eating habits in their families, partners, and friends reduce their meat intake and shift their own diets toward healthier, unprocessed plant foods to set a good example for their loved ones. Because plant-based diets can improve so many components of well-being, they can suit anyone and everyone, as long as they are executed in a mindful manner.

Although nutrition science is a rapidly evolving field, research continues to corroborate the findings of *The China Study*: that increasing consumption of vegetables, fruit, whole grains, nuts, seeds, and plant-based proteins, as well as reducing meat intake and refined food consumption, can help prevent and treat a wide range of conditions, including type 2 diabetes, hypercholesterolemia, dyslipidemia (high triglycerides), hypertension, heart and fatty liver disease, certain cancers, some neurological diseases, hormonal imbalances, infertility, symptoms of PMS and PCOS, and psycho-emotional disorders such as depression, anxiety, and ADHD. Of course, not everyone reaps all of these benefits, but mounting evidence suggests that a plant-based lifestyle can do wonders for many people suffering myriad illnesses.

A noteworthy 2014 study by González et al., for instance, showed that even a mild increase in vegetable intake coupled with a reduction in animal-sourced food consumption yielded health improvements. In this study, the researchers developed a provegetarian score—a rating system which compared the quantity of fruits and vegetables people consumed to how much meat they consumed—based on repeated dietary measures in omnivorous Spanish adults with a high risk of cardiovascular disease. Plant foods were weighted positively while animal foods were weighted negatively, meaning the higher the score, the more plant-based the subject's diet. The authors found that the higher the provegetarian score, the lower the risk of mortality from all causes, including cardiovascular disease. The study was even more nuanced because it tiered the scores, comparing very low provegetarian scores to low scores, moderate scores, and high scores, finding that as scores increased incrementally, so did health benefits. The takeaway? As vegetable intake increased and meat consumption decreased, so did health benefits, and vice versa. This study is one of many indicating that the health benefits of a plant-based diet are real and profound, and can be achieved even with the inclusion of some animal products. You do not need to go to the extreme and become vegan or even fully vegetarian to get results.

The Environment

We're all familiar with how global warming is jeopardizing our planet. In the past two years alone, we've seen the Australia and California wildfires, floods in Europe and China, earthquake in Haiti, Hurricanes Harvey and Ida, and melting glaciers in Greenland and Iceland.

According to an overwhelming majority of climate scientists and the Intergovernmental Panel on Climate Change (IPCC) of the United Nations, human activity on both the individual and collective level is the main cause of global warming. Culpable activities cited by the UN include the growing use of coal and overall industrialization in China and India, large-scale agriculture, deforestation, extreme population growth, overuse of automobiles, air travel, heating and cooling systems, and importantly, the amount of animal products we consume. Each of these undertakings contribute to the release of harmful greenhouse gases—CO_2, methane, and nitric oxide—which interfere with the atmosphere and add to global warming.

I am not here to preach about climate change; I simply want to provide facts about the impact food production has on the environment. So, let's take a closer look. Animal agriculture and food production together, which support our meat- and dairy-eating habits and drive the consequential chain reaction of events responsible for many facets of environmental damage, produce approximately a quarter of greenhouse gas emissions in the form of nitrous oxide and methane (carbon emissions are allocated to the energy sector). They are the second greatest contributor of human-made greenhouse gas emissions after fossil fuels, and also the leading cause of deforestation, water use and contamination, and air pollution. On the subject of deforestation, animal agriculture is responsible for 80 percent of forestry burning, which releases more carbon into the atmosphere than all exploitable fossil fuel reserves. The clearing of forests also eliminates the planet's ability to absorb carbon, which is the job of trees. As for water, approximately 70 percent of fresh water evaporated or removed from the watershed is used for food production. (A watershed—also known as a drainage basin or catchment—is an area of land that drains all the streams and rainfall to a common outlet like a reservoir, bay, or stream channel.) Together, these effects make animal agriculture the largest contributor to biodiversity loss globally.

Research has identified meat as the food whose production has the greatest impact on greenhouse gases and land use. Production of 1,000 kilocalories of lamb or beef generates fourteen kilograms and ten kilograms, respectively, of greenhouse gas emissions, compared to 1,000 kilocalories of tofu or lentils, which generates one kilogram and three kilograms, respectively. Furthermore, producing a single serving of beef requires 1,211 liters of water and a single serving of pork 469 liters, compared to the 220 liters it takes to produce one serving of dried beans, the 57 it takes for a serving of tofu, and the 30 liters required for tomato production.

Although these statistics may seem insurmountable, the good news is that as an individual, you can help reduce these emissions, as well as water, land, and energy use, merely by decreasing your consumption of meat by even a small amount. A 2018 study modeled the effects of different diet scenarios in 150 countries in all regions of the world and found several notable results. One conclusion was that the widespread adoption of plant-based eating patterns, which reduce animal-sourced products anywhere between 25 and 100 percent, would reduce global environmental impact, nutrient deficiencies, and mortality. Another was that four specific nutritionally balanced, plant-based eating patterns could also reduce impacts on environmental and human health globally. Those four diets are the ones I am focusing on in this book: flexitarian (limited red meat, moderate animal-sourced foods, plant foods); pescatarian (meat replaced with fish, moderate animal-sourced foods, plant foods); vegetarian (no meat, moderate animal-sourced foods, plant foods); and vegan (no animal-sourced foods, plant foods).

Since 2014, research and awareness about sustainable diets, a concept that combines environmental and health concerns, has expanded. Systematic reviews have suggested that reductions in the environmental impacts of food production are generally proportional to reductions in animal-sourced foods, which in turn have a positive effect on health. Interestingly, the approaches that included healthy eating as a motivator were more successful than those focused only on reducing environmental pressures.

Animal Welfare

Whereas climate change pushes some folks toward plant-based eating, others are equally or more concerned about animal welfare. According to the Humane Society International, over eighty billion animals worldwide are slaughtered for food every year, mostly on factory farms. Factory farming is the main mechanism of industrialized food production; it is how the majority of red meat, pork, and chicken ends up on our tables. Unfortunately, the industrialized processing of animal-based products involves practices many believe are incredibly cruel toward animals. From the time they are born until the time they are killed, livestock and other animals consumed as food are separated from their mothers, kept in confined solitary spaces, handled violently, fed unsanitary food, subjected to intense stress such as electric shocks, and injected with hormones and antibiotics (which ultimately end up in us).

But not all animal-sourced food production involves such practices, and you need not feel guilty about the desire to keep some animal products in your diet, even if you're going plant-based. If you enjoy meat and want to continue eating it, there are healthier, more compassionate, and more sustainable ways of obtaining your animal-based food products. You can eat locally farmed, organic, pasture-raised, and grass-fed meat, dairy, eggs, pork, and chicken, and stay away from animal products that are highly processed.

Foods That Fit...Or Don't

The first step to adopting a plant-based diet is to learn about common categories of food that complement fruits and vegetables in a plant-based diet. The second is to decide whether you want to include them in your eating pattern. The benefits of incorporating a robust variety of fresh fruits and vegetables in any diet are incontrovertible, yet conflicting research and conflated media stories have propagated numerous myths about the foods highlighted in this section, leaving people misinformed and dubious—often for the wrong reasons—about whether to incorporate them into their diet. The foods that I've found elicit the most questions and concerns, particularly by those trying to eat in a more plant-based way, are soy, legumes, eggs, dairy, fish, meat, and processed goods.

Soy

"Where Do We Stand on Soy?" headlines a 2018 CNN article. "Is Soy Good or Bad for you? Here's the Science-Backed Answer," leads another 2020 piece in *Good Housekeeping*. From hard news to lifestyle publications, the debate on soy is ongoing, and the science on soy, like many foods, is often misunderstood or misinterpreted.

Here's the truth: save for if you're allergic to soy or have a medical reason to avoid eating it (e.g. hypothyroidism, IBS), this food can be a terrific and nutritious addition to your diet with many health benefits. For instance, soy is a staple of many Asian diets, which are considered some of the healthiest eating patterns on the planet. The traditional Okinawan diet, for instance, includes about eight times more soy than that of the typical American diet and Okinawa was ranked among *National Geographic* fellow Dan Buettner's "Blue Zones." (Blue Zones are places in the world Buettner identified as home to the greatest number of centenarians—the longest-living and healthiest people on Earth.)

The science on soy shows that its health benefits are manifold and outweigh its minimal possible risks. First, soy contains isoflavones, a class of phytoestrogen. (Phytoestrogens are plant-derived compounds found in a wide variety of foods that have many health benefits but are also known to be weak estrogen agonists/antagonists and potential endocrine disrupters.) Some studies associate these compounds with the prevention of bone loss; improved sleep quality; lower depression; lower risk of menopausal symptoms like hot flashes; reduced risk of cardiovascular disease, obesity, metabolic syndrome, type 2 diabetes, and brain function disorders; and reduced risks of several cancers, including colon, stomach, prostate, rectal, and breast. Second, soy is high in calcium, which, in addition to being key for bone health, could be an additional regulator of breast cancer cell proliferation. Third, soy contains a lot of fiber, including an important type called pectic polysaccharides. Pectic polysaccharides regulate proteins that may otherwise cause cell death in the colon and that are essential for any healthy diet because they reduce cholesterol, blood glucose, diabetes, and risk of heart disease and cancer. Furthermore, intestinal bacteria ferment and degrade this fiber, which helps normalize the overall gut microbiome. Finally, soybeans are a good source of protein, unsaturated fatty acids, B vitamins, iron, zinc, and other bioactive compounds, which make edamame, tempeh, tofu, and natto excellent food choices.

The issue with soy that seems to draw the most negative attention pertains to its connection to hormones and fertility. Many people believe that the phytoestrogens in soy can reduce fertility, because some studies have shown that, in excess, phytoestrogens can signal the body that the estrogen environment is high, which in turn can cause it to stop producing estrogen (in a negative feedback loop). Estrogen is necessary for the process of ovulation and pregnancy to begin because it initiates the cascade of fertility hormones to take off (gonadotropin, FSH, and LH). Thus, a low estrogen environment due to the presence of phytoestrogens could prevent the release of other fertility hormones.

The research, however, only suggests a possible association between phytoestrogens and infertility if a person ingests more than one hundred milligrams of isoflavones a day—an amount drastically higher than the typical human consumes, and which could potentially, but not necessarily, induce the body to think estrogen is high. Here is some context in which to frame this: the average isoflavone consumption in the US is approximately 2.5 milligrams per day, while traditional Asian diets, which are higher in soy, contain approximately ten to twenty-five milligrams of isoflavones per day. As there are about twenty-five milligrams of isoflavones in one cup or serving of soymilk made from whole soybeans, one hundred milligrams would be equivalent to four cups of soymilk.

So, how much soy is safe to eat with regards to fertility concerns? Studies to date suggest that anywhere from one to two servings (cups) of soy per day is benign (two servings is fifteen grams of soy protein or fifty milligrams of isoflavones), provides the above-mentioned benefits, and poses no risk of infertility. Those seeking soy's cholesterol-lowering capabilities, however, might have to increase their daily intake of soy protein to twenty-five grams, which is still significantly under the prospective daily limit of one hundred milligrams of isoflavones.

For similar reasons, studies also suggest that the phytoestrogens in soy could aggravate endometriosis. Women who suffer from endometriosis often overproduce estrogen to begin with; since phytoestrogens can bind to estrogen receptors, the assumption is that they could signal the body to elevate estrogen levels even further, which in turn could thicken the uterus. While an association between phytoestrogens and endometriosis requires further research, many studies, in fact, already indicate the opposite effect of phytoestrogens on endometriosis. These studies show that because phytoestrogens can prevent actual estrogen from binding to receptors in high-estrogen environments (because phytoestrogens bind first), they could in fact have anti-estrogenic effects (they are also weaker than estrogens), thereby reducing the risk of endometriosis. The evidence of soy's effect on endometriosis is inconclusive and highly dependent on individual genetics, age, metabolism, gut microflora, antibiotic use, underlying conditions, environment (variety, harvest, food processing, cooking, and growth locations of foods), and how much soy one consumes.

The most definitive evidence on the adverse effects of phytoestrogens applies to their interaction with the thyroid. If you have hypothyroidism and are taking medications for the condition, your doctor might advise you to stay away from soy because it can prevent the absorption of thyroid medication, as well as uptake of some of the iodine needed to make thyroid hormones.

While some people should indeed be cautious about soy consumption for the above-mentioned rationales (and if you suffer from IBS, soy could also be a culprit and you might try an elimination diet to see if removing it alleviates your discomfort), there are good reasons for most to start or continue eating food from this category in moderation. The best way to make the decision about whether to consume soy is to weigh the pros and cons in the context of your particular health status with your doctor or dietician.

Legumes

Legumes are edible, nutritious seeds in the form of pods, such as beans, lentils, chickpeas, peanuts, and alfalfa sprouts. Like soy, they are another food group that sparks controversy, because fad diets such as Whole30 and Paleo swear they do no good. I can assure you, however, that demonizing these powerhouses is misguided, because a large body of evidence illuminates their health benefits, which generally outweigh their potential costs. Yet despite the science, only about 8 percent of US adults eat legumes on any given day.

If you're going plant-based, here are some reasons you might want to eat legumes. They are a rich source of protein, fiber, carbohydrates, B vitamins, iron, copper, magnesium, manganese, zinc, and phosphorous. They are naturally low in total fat, practically free of saturated fat, and cholesterol-free. They have a low glycemic index, which means they do not cause a fast insulin spike. Finally, legumes contain lectins, which are antioxidants that slow the digestion of carbohydrates and can kill cancer cells. For all of these reasons, many studies support legumes as a critical part of a healthy eating pattern, highlighting that they lower the risk of type 2 diabetes, hyperlipidemia (because they lower low-density lipoproteins, or LDLs), and hypertension (because potassium, magnesium, and fiber all have a positive effect on blood pressure). Moreover, for those hoping to shave off a few pounds, these gems could also have the potential to assist in weight reduction; their high fiber content lends to feeling more satisfied, which could result in eating less.

Given the above, you might be wondering why so many trendy diets, and individuals who follow them, are so quick to eliminate legumes from their meal plans. Let me explain. The concern about legumes stems from the fact that they contain anti-nutrients such as phytates and lectins. (Anti-nutrients are natural compounds found in many plant- and animal-derived foods that can bind to the cell walls of the digestive tract, which can in turn disrupt the breakdown and absorption of nutrients while affecting the growth and action of intestinal flora.) Theoretically, phytates and lectins could decrease the absorption of iron, zinc, magnesium, calcium, and phosphorous. It is unknown, however, to what extent nutrient loss actually occurs due to these anti-nutrients for a couple of reasons: individual metabolisms cause variation and the amount and effect of phytates and lectins highly depends on how one prepares, cooks, and eats their legumes. For instance, soaking, boiling, or sprouting legumes before consuming them—and we rarely eat them otherwise—reduces, removes, and deactivates anti-nutrients, rendering them harmless.

If you still have doubts about anti-nutrients in legumes, here is another point of information that may allay your skepticism: phytates and lectins might exert an effect on nutrients in one meal but not the next. In other words, too many legumes in one sitting could in theory increase the risk of poor nutrient absorption, but the same quantity would not have any overall effect if spread out over other meals. Thus, if you eat a balanced diet with normal portion sizes (no more than half a cup of legumes per meal), you should have no reason to worry. And here's another interesting piece of research: studies on vegetarians, who could be at risk of nutrient deficiencies due to diets high in plant foods containing anti-nutrients, show that they do not generally lack iron or zinc, which leads scientists to presume that the body might adjust to the presence of nutrient antagonists by increasing the gut's absorptive capacity of the affected minerals.

You can tell I am a fan of legumes because of their rich health profile, but, like any food, they aren't for everyone. High in bloat-causing fiber, lentils, black beans, chickpeas, and other such foods can wreak havoc on the digestive systems of those with IBS, Crohn's disease, ulcerative colitis, diverticulosis, and other gut-related issues (adding baking soda during preparation is a key secret to reducing potential bloating and gas). If you suffer from discomfort due to legumes, however, before you simply stop eating them, consult a dietician with whom you can work to discover if there are certain varieties and ways you can eat them (e.g., minimal amounts or puréed) or if you must eliminate them all together.

Eggs

Having taken on two controversial groups of plant-derived foods, it's time to dive into animal-sourced products that also fit into a plant-based eating pattern, but are often approached with uncertainty. Swearing off animal-sourced foods entirely is unappealing and unsustainable for a good portion of the population, like the many of us who love a plate of fluffy scrambled eggs, a perfectly poached egg atop a slice of whole grain avocado toast, or a sating bowl of shakshuka. Not to mention all the foods that eggs turn up in, such as baked goods and casseroles.

Including eggs in your plant-based diet has many upsides. Eggs are cheap, low in calories (about seventy calories per egg), and high in protein. They also contain a variety of other nutrients including folate, riboflavin, selenium, choline, vitamin B-12, vitamin K, and vitamin D. Eggs can enhance the bioavailability of antioxidants lutein and zeaxanthin, which fight disease-causing free radicals. Furthermore, despite common thinking based on obsolete research, most healthy people do not need to worry that eggs will elevate their cholesterol. The latest research concludes that: 1) Dietary cholesterol (cholesterol in food) does not adversely affect the body's total cholesterol levels or risk of cardiovascular disease and 2) The consumption of one egg per day, or up to seven a week, is perfectly acceptable for those who are not genetically predisposed to elevated plasma cholesterol and who do not have type 2 diabetes (which interferes with cholesterol transport). Those with diabetes should consider eating less than three eggs per week.

DEBUNKING THE MYTH OF THE "EVIL EGG"

Are you still convinced that eggs have no business in a healthy diet because you remember hearing that even half an egg a day is bad for you? I get your concerns, but let me give some context. Many of the studies that gave rise to this popular thinking were done in the 1970s and were not intervention studies (meaning they did not compare the test group to a control group). These studies, which were observational studies, analyzed participants over time who ate eggs and examined how the eggs affected them, without comparing them to subjects who did not eat eggs. (Comparative studies, also known as intervention studies, are the gold standard in nutrition science; observational studies are always therefore taken with a grain of salt.) Second, they did not consider what participants ate in addition to eggs (e.g. bacon, white toast, butter, hash browns), which would highly influence all risk factors. Finally, the authors failed to examine with what participants substituted eggs if they didn't eat them, which could have had positive or negative effects on outcomes. These oversights not only led the way for the current research, which has cleared the egg's reputation, but also gave birth to today's United States Department of Agriculture 2015–2020 guidelines, which do not set limits on the amount of dietary cholesterol one can consume.

If you love eggs or feel you need them to meet your protein and other nutrient requirements, I hope you'll eat them because, for most people, they really do fit into a healthy, strong, and nutritious plant-based lifestyle. Just be mindful about from where you're purchasing them (local farms that sell pasture-raised eggs from grass-fed chickens are best), how you're preparing them (cook them in olive or canola oil as opposed to butter to reduce saturated fat intake and get the incredibly healthy monounsaturated fatty acids instead), how many you're eating, and with what you're eating them. Salt, sugar, fat, and excess calories in highly processed foods such as ham, sausage, and biscuits commonly creep in as complements to eggs, so choose healthier alternatives such as avocado, spinach, fresh fruit, 100 percent whole grain toast, flourless seed bread, or tortillas made with nut and legume-based flours.

On the other hand, if you're thinking about going plant-based for animal welfare or health reasons, you may choose to avoid eggs. Unfortunately, chickens are treated no better than cows or pigs—unless you buy local, pasture-raised, grass-fed, organic eggs, which are sourced from chickens that are treated more humanely than those produced on factory farms.

Dairy

One of the foods clients and friends most commonly ask me about is dairy: What do you think about milk? Should I cut it out? What about for my kids? What's the stuff about hormones? How about acne? What about cheese? Do you eat it? What are your thoughts on milk substitutes?

If you're determined to eliminate all animal products from your diet, whether for health, the environment, or animal welfare, it's time to say goodbye to dairy. But for the rest of us, while dairy is often vilified by diet culture, in moderation, it can be a nutritionally powerful part of any diet, including plant-based ones.

Dairy is replete with vital nutrients including calcium, vitamin D, vitamin B-12, and high-quality protein, which are crucial for bone and muscle health from childhood throughout life, protecting against ailments such as rickets, sarcopenia, osteoporosis, and osteopenia. In addition, although research is mixed, numerous studies show that dairy is associated with fewer incidences of cardiometabolic disease, including childhood obesity, type 2 diabetes, cardiac events such as arrythmias and heart valve disease, strokes, chronic inflammation, and several types of cancer (colorectal, bladder, gastric, and breast cancer). Moreover, this may be surprising, but studies show that in adults, dairy can support weight loss and improve body composition. This is because milk proteins such as whey contain branched-chain amino acids like leucine, which assist with muscle protein synthesis while reducing fat mass.

If you enjoy dairy and rely on it to ensure the intake of essential nutrients, I encourage you to understand the latest guidelines. The American Heart Association recommends non-fat or low-fat dairy, which studies show have an inverse relationship with hypertension and stroke. Coupled with this evidence, newer research indicates that if you have a well-balanced healthy diet with controlled saturated fat, salt, sugar, cholesterol, and calorie intake, you can also enjoy full-fat dairy products in reasonable quantities without having to worry about weight gain or increased risk of chronic disease. (This is because people often consume more low- and non-fat dairy products than regular ones, increasing their calorie and sugar intake, which in conjunction with other poor diet choices can reduce and even nullify their beneficial effects.) Furthermore, some studies support the intake of dairy foods such as cheese and fermented products like yogurt and kefir, in light of evidence showing they can reduce coronary artery disease and positively affect gut health due to their probiotic content. (Probiotics are live organisms present in certain foods. They are associated with enhanced gut health because of how they interact with the trillions of other bacteria in our intestinal microbiome as well as our brain, organs, and other body systems. Probiotics can suppress pathogens, modulate our immune systems, reduce systemic inflammation, and stimulate epithelial cell proliferation, differentiation, and fortification of the intestinal barrier.)

But dairy isn't for everyone. Lactose intolerance is a real and prevalent condition. If you suffer from abdominal discomfort, gas, diarrhea, or vomiting after consuming dairy, it's possible that—like 65 percent of the world's population—your body doesn't produce lactase, the main enzyme that digests lactose. If you have symptoms like the above, don't wait and wonder. Go to your doctor and get a hydrogen breath or a blood glucose test to see if you are lactose intolerant. If your results are positive, you can reduce or eliminate your consumption of dairy, or stay away from forms and quantities of it that trigger your symptoms.

LACTOSE INTOLERANCE

Many lactose-intolerant individuals can tolerate certain quantities and types of dairy such as a glass of milk, a scoop of ice cream, and especially hard cheese and fermented dairy products like yogurt and kefir. Why? Regarding milk and ice cream, reactions are often dose responsive (which means that symptoms only occur at certain quantitative thresholds). As for cheese and fermented products like yogurt, the former contains negligible lactose, and the latter has a form of lactose (with bacterial lactase) that the body digests more easily than the lactose in milk.

Another reason you might choose to abstain from consuming dairy is if you are allergic to any of a number of milk proteins. Casein and whey are the two most common proteins to which people are allergic. Like lactose intolerance, there are tests for these allergies. If you are indeed allergic to one or both, it's possible you'll need to avoid cow, goat, sheep, and buffalo milk.

Finally, if your incentive for becoming dairy-free is that you're concerned about hormones (growth hormone IGF-1) and antibiotics that end up in your body potentially causing acne or increasing your risk of certain types of cancer (e.g., prostate cancer), or because you're an animal rights or sustainability advocate, it's totally legitimate to reduce or eliminate it from your diet. Dairy can be inflammatory and isn't necessary for optimal well-being; you can get all the nutrients it provides from other foods (e.g., dark leafy greens, soy, legumes). Just be aware that the nutrient profiles of plant-based milk substitutes are completely different from that of milk and cannot be considered equal alternatives. Though few studies to date have compared dairy to its substitutes, the current science illuminates things to consider when choosing your alternatives: 1) Soy is the only plant-based milk that contains a similar amount of high-quality protein to milk. 2) The nutrient profiles of milk substitutes vary considerably depending on how they have been processed and fortified. Many have added sugar, vegetable oils, the inflammatory agent carrageenan, and are more caloric than regular dairy. Though they may be fortified with some vitamins and minerals, they can be deficient in others present in regular milk. 3) There are cases of severe nutritional deficiencies in children due to inappropriate consumption of plant-based drinks. (For more on alternative dairy beverages, go to pages 110–111.)

DOES DAIRY CAUSE ACNE?

For a long time, it has been thought that the Western diet, and dairy specifically, may cause acne. The theory behind dairy and acne is based on the fact that hormones injected into cows and/or milk-derived amino acids may promote insulin secretion and induce hepatic insulin-like growth factor-1 (IGF-1) synthesis. Studies suggest that IGF-1 may be a primary driver of acne because it stimulates the growth of cohesive follicular epithelial cells that don't shed correctly, and which drive sebum production and inflammation. But whereas several studies show a correlation between dairy and acne, these studies are limited and the evidence inconclusive. One recent systematic review and meta-analysis, for instance, concluded that the odds ratio, which measures the possibility that dairy is associated with acne, suggests that any dairy such as milk, yogurt, and cheese, was associated with an increased odds ratio for acne in individuals aged seven to thirty years old. In addition, this study showed that the more milk subjects drank per week, the greater the odds ratio (1.24 for two to six glasses of milk per week, 1.41 for one glass per day, and 1.43 for greater than two glasses per day). As for full-fat milk versus low-fat and skim milk, this study indicated that the association between dairy and acne increased for skim milk, possibly because people drank more of it. Finally, this study also showed that cheese had a higher odds ratio for its association with acne than other type of dairy. So, here's the catch: despite the results, the authors indicate bias in the study and discuss that there are many other potential causes of acne—including diet and genetics—making it hard to single out and determine causation by any one component.

Fish

Although fish is perhaps less controversial than the other food categories discussed thus far, there are some common uncertainties to be addressed. Two questions that frequently arise are: Why is fish distinguished from meat? And why do some people eat fish but not meat?

Meat, by definition, is the "flesh of an animal (especially a mammal) as food," whereas fish is "flesh of fish used for food." With this in mind, some people justify eating fish, but not meat, arguing that fish are cold-blooded, hairless, and do not feel pain (this is debatable). Others, however, eat fish—but not meat—for religious reasons. And yet others, like me, refrain from eating meat but still eat fish for what I call aesthetic reasons (taste, texture, mouthfeel, appearance, smell), along with the health benefits, and provision of variety in a diet. Then, there are those who do not differentiate between the two and eat both, or neither, considering fish to be meat because they are animals, period.

The strongest argument in favor of eating fish but not meat is that numerous studies show it is much healthier than meat. Unlike meat, evidence illustrates that fish consumption can lower risk of cardiovascular and chronic disease, while it has no effect on cancer. Second, fish is noted for its high levels of protein, vitamin D, vitamin B2 (riboflavin), calcium, phosphorous, iron, zinc, iodine, magnesium, potassium, and vitamin B-12. Third, fish is famous for its high content of healthy omega-3 fatty acids. According to the USDA, eating fish, particularly varieties high in omega-3s, at least twice a week (each serving would be approximately four ounces), appears to reduce the incidence of cardiac events, especially sudden ones like heart failure, stroke, and arrhythmias, because they combat inflammation, reduce triglycerides, lower blood pressure, decrease blood clotting, and keep the heart beating at a steady clip.

Despite these benefits, there are also reasons to be cautious about fish consumption. As with livestock, raising fish for food adversely affects the welfare of entire species and environmental sustainability. Like land animals, fish are often bred, fed, and treated in unnatural and cruel ways. Farmed fish can be crowded into small, unclean, and bound areas, fed chemicals such as dioxins and polychlorinated biphenyls (PCBs), and killed in ways believed to be particularly inhumane. Wild fish are also exposed to toxins from industrial runoff that pollutes the oceans and seas. Certain types of fish for example, including king mackerel, tuna steak, swordfish, tilefish, marlin, and Chilean sea bass, are high in mercury and other potentially poisonous chemicals. Finally, overfishing taxes marine systems, destroying coral and kelp forests and divesting ocean ecosystems of their equilibrium, while bycatch, which refers to accidentally catching animals other than the intended fish—including turtles, dolphins, and seabirds—threatens these populations, as well as those of the fish intended to be caught. Although bycatch is a lesser-publicized issue than some of the others in aquaculture, it is a serious problem and threat to our planet.

Meat

While the science showing the negative effects of meat consumption on health, the environment, and animal welfare is clear, we still have an extraordinarily difficult time jettisoning it from our diets: a 2018 USDA report forecasts that the average meat-eating American will have access to and consume approximately 222.2 pounds of red meat and poultry alone in a year!

Why? Meat is readily available in most of the world, affordable, and ingrained as a meal staple in many cultures. In addition, people enjoy the unique taste and texture of it, as well as the experience of preparing it, from grilling hamburgers and hotdogs with family and friends on the fourth of July, to massaging a steak with a marinade, to the family rituals around cooking a turkey for Thanksgiving. Meat is also a very high source of protein, iron, and vitamin B-12, all of which the body needs and craves. Yet despite the appeal of meat, as discussed earlier, the numbers of people considering reducing or foregoing it are rising for several reasons.

Climate weighs heavy on many, and meat, more than any other food we consume, is the greatest contributor to our planet's ill health. On average, producing meat (and dairy) is far more resource-intensive than producing plant-based protein, requiring eleven times more fossil fuel energy than grain-based protein. Furthermore, red meat production is one of the most highly inefficient systems, with an estimated ratio of kilocalories of energy expended to kilocalories of protein generating a fifty-seven-to-one ratio for lamb and a forty-to-one ratio for beef. Due to the increasing demand for meat (because the population is growing and humans love to eat it), food production systems are under such incredible stress that researchers predict they will not be able to sustain future population growth, especially when simultaneously contending with the negative effects of climate change.

You may also be reconsidering meat intake after reading that many meat varieties including red, processed, and white meat contain high amounts of saturated fat, hormones, and antibiotics, which evidence consistently demonstrates are associated with a higher risk of heart disease, several types of cancer (stomach, bladder, breast, colorectal), and type 2 diabetes. Perhaps you've come across articles in the news about processed meat as even more problematic than unprocessed meat because it contains nitrites and nitrates, which correlate with an increased risk of heart disease and cancer, especially colon cancer.

When it comes to health and diets, however, it doesn't have to be all or nothing; moderation is an option. Two very influential, large, and long-term studies, which analyzed risk factors including nutrition for chronic diseases, showed that replacing one serving of red meat per day with fish, poultry, legumes, nuts, low-fat dairy, or whole grains lowered the risk of premature death by 7 to 19 percent. The authors found similar results when they looked at how swapping small amounts of meat with the above alternatives affected type 2 diabetes. Research further indicates that simply reducing your meat consumption to low or moderate amounts (no more than two to three portions per week totaling two to eighteen ounces) has the potential to decrease your total chronic disease risk, while still allowing you to enjoy and reap the nutritional benefits of it (e.g. protein, iron, B-12). The bottom line? If you like meat and want to keep it in your diet, you can, just do so mindfully.

Processed Food

As with meat, research is consistent on whether we should include processed food, snacks, and sweets in our diets. Evidence clarifies it is essential to minimize our intake of these foods for all the causes covered thus far—our health, the environment, and animal welfare. The packaged food industry thrives on using salt, sugar, and fat to hook the consumer and achieve corporate gains, even though its products end up devastating those things that matter to us most. According to the Dietary Guidelines for Americans 2020–2025, we consume more than 1,000 extra milligrams of sodium than recommended (3,393 milligrams compared to 2,300 milligrams for the average adult), mostly from commercially processed food. The top sources of sodium are sandwiches at 21 percent (think deli meat, mayonnaise, cheese); rice, pasta, and other mixed grain-based dishes at 8 percent; and pre-made vegetables at 7 percent. The same goes for added sugar, of which we consume more than twice the recommended daily amount (13 percent as opposed to 7 percent), with the top sources including sugar-sweetened beverages at 24 percent, desserts and sweet snacks at 19 percent, and coffee and tea drinks at 11 percent (think added milk, cream, whipped cream, and syrups). When it comes to saturated fat, the top category is again sandwiches at 21 percent; desserts and sweet snacks at 11 percent; and rice, pasta, and other mixed grain dishes at 7 percent.

I understand that with life's limitations of time, affordability, and access, it can be very difficult if not impossible for many people to reduce and even eliminate processed food. That said, I want you to have the knowledge so that to the extent you *can* reduce and avoid these foods, you will. The easiest way to work on this is to prepare your food at home as frequently as possible, using whole, organic ingredients. Avocado, egg, and tuna salad toasts you prepare in your kitchen (see recipes in Lunch Mains starting on page 156) are healthy, easy-to-make alternatives to sandwiches with processed meat you would buy at the deli, convenience store, or fast-food joint. Homemade chocolate chip cookies (see recipe on page 277) are not equivalent to bagged and boxed chocolate chip cookies. Water, black coffee, and plain tea are always better choices than soda, juice, and coffees and teas we buy sweetened with milk, sugar, and whipped cream. You don't need to deprive yourself of the occasional treat. While I am extremely mindful about the detriments of consistently consuming commercially processed food, and encourage you to be cautious too, I confess to eating ice cream, drinking a diet coke, and indulging in some chips occasionally.

Not All Plant-Based Diets Are Created Equal

Now that you know the pros and cons of controversial foods that can be part of your plant-based lifestyle, let's tackle implementing the right diet for you. But first, I want you to keep one critical piece of information in mind: the key to successfully adopting any plant-based diet is to substitute animal-derived and processed products with whole, organic, nutrient-dense foods such as fruits, vegetables, legumes, whole grains, nuts, seeds, and plant-based proteins rather than with refined carbohydrates, sugar, salt, and excessive amounts of plant-based saturated fats. If your goal is to improve your health, becoming plant-based in the latter manner could maintain your condition as is, or even make it worse, increasing your susceptibility to malnourishment, chronic disease, and mortality. Studies for instance have shown that non-celiacs who become gluten-free as part of a plant-based diet and others who implement an "unhealthy plant-based diet" can be more susceptible to type 2 diabetes and coronary heart disease because they end up eating less fiber, and more cream, butter, sugar, and refined carbohydrates. Through an in-depth look at the four plant-based diets introduced earlier and a step-by-step guide to executing each one, Part Two of this book will show you how to avoid these outcomes so that you can adopt a plant-based lifestyle in a healthful and nutritious manner.

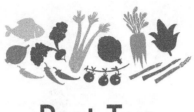

Part Two

THE GUIDE

Which Diet Is Best for Me?

I am sure that you, like myself and so many others, struggle with food and your lifestyle around it. I also know that diet culture preys on our weaknesses by putting forth seductively simple plans that purport to be the solutions for everyone. But as science has progressed, the notion that one diet can solve every individual's weight, health, and spiritual problems has been proven false. The most recent and promising research for the future of "dieting" is in fact focused on personalized nutrition, "tailored nutritional recommendations aimed at the promotion, maintenance of health and prevention against diseases." According to the 2018 study "Challenges in Personalized Nutrition and Health," this approach to nutrition takes into account the following aspects of each human's unique makeup: distinct responses to individualized, food-derived nutrients that arise due to the interaction between nutrients and biological processes; internal interactions between an individual's genetics, microbiome, and metabolome; and external factors such as dietary habits and physical activity.

I am an ardent believer in customized diets, so the purpose of this guide is to provide you with several tips for how you can implement a personalized plant-based lifestyle. My aim is fourfold: 1) to teach you how to transition to a plant-based lifestyle effectively and nutritiously; 2) to introduce you to four plant-based eating patterns—flexitarian, pescatarian, vegetarian, and vegan; 3) to assist you in determining how far into the plant-based lifestyle you want and need to go in order to achieve your goals (i.e. which eating pattern is right for you at any given time in your life); and 4) to assist you in developing eating habits and behaviors that can last a lifetime.

I have selected the flexitarian, pescatarian, vegetarian, and vegan diets for several reasons. The study of the correlation between diet and the environment in 150 countries discussed in Part One (see page 9) suggests that if adopted, these four diets—which are nutritionally balanced eating patterns—improve nutrient levels and decrease diet-related premature deaths in all

29

regions, while leading to reductions in environmental impacts in high- and middle-income countries (by alleviating stress from factory farming and supporting more ethical farming practices). They also reduce the suffering of animals. Finally, these diets not only enhance overall health and well-being, but they are also achievable because they provide a wide range of options to accommodate individual lifestyles and preferences.

As you proceed through this guide, I would like you to think of the eating patterns as ranked from least to most restrictive with flexitarian being the most expansive followed by pescatarian, vegetarian, and lastly, vegan. If you are new to plant-based eating, I suggest you follow the diets in the order I present them for the best and most sustainable results. This progressive approach will allow you to check in with yourself as you move through each eating pattern so that you can decide if you have gone far enough, or if you want to continue to the next diet. In other words, if you transition from being an omnivore to a flexitarian by reducing red and processed meat and are comfortable with that, you can stop there. But if you have had success with the flexitarian lifestyle and are interested in eliminating meat all together, you will be ready to transition to a pescatarian eating pattern with much greater ease than if you were to jump directly from a meat-heavy omnivorous diet to a lifestyle that only allows for fish. Similarly, becoming vegetarian is much easier if you are pescatarian first than if you transition from being flexitarian. The same governing principle— the larger the leap between diets, the greater the challenge with compliance and sustainability will be—applies across the board. (The lack of attention to this concept is a top reason fad diets don't work.)

Remember: no one of these diets is inherently better than another. So, if at any point in time you're thinking, "If I don't make it to vegan, I am a failure," think again. If a vegan diet—or any of the others—seems unappealing, unsustainable, unattainable, or if trying it makes you miserable, it doesn't mean that you are undisciplined or incapable. It is more likely that the eating pattern is just not right for you.

Before we start our journey through each individual diet, here are some guidelines that apply to all four eating patterns, including how to transition from one to the next, the importance of assessment, tips and strategies that pertain to eating environments, the significance of finding a supportive community, the necessity of incorporating exercise into your life, the importance of mindfulness, and the need for self-nurturing.

How to Transition

When it comes to refining one's eating habits, I always advise my clients to have a plan with the goal of longevity. A little contemplation goes a long way and makes life a whole lot easier by helping avoid unforeseen obstacles to healthy intentions. Whichever eating pattern you start with, when you decide you are ready to progress from one diet to the next, plan for a six-week transition period during which you will focus on reducing, substituting, and eliminating the "Transition Foods" that pertain to each plan. This does not mean you will be eating less or hungry, but that you will be replacing nutrient-poor foods with nutrient-rich foods, which will ultimately be equally if not more filling and satisfying. For instance, if you are moving from being an omnivore to a flexitarian, you will reduce red and processed meat and substitute them with white meat, fish, dairy, eggs, and plant foods; if you are transitioning from flexitarian to pescatarian, you will reduce white meat and replace it with fish, dairy, eggs, and plant foods; if you are transitioning from pescatarian to vegetarian, you will reduce fish and substitute it with eggs, dairy, and plant foods; and if you are moving from vegetarian to vegan, you will reduce eggs and dairy and add more plant proteins to your meal plan. For all eating patterns, you will also work on reducing and eliminating processed foods as well as modifying your consumption of foods high in sodium, sugar, and saturated fat. The transition period will be followed by two weeks of honing and maintenance.

A brief explanation and timeline, which applies to all the diets, is outlined below. Though I am using hypothetical meals to explain how to transition, the overarching principles apply to foods you are in fact eating and several of the recipes speak to the recipe section of this book. If you need longer for your transition than allotted, do not worry. Read the Assessment section (page 39) and you will see that you can extend your timeline. Again, the idea is not that you will be eating less, but that you will be eating healthier and feeling better with more energy and focus, and less stress.

PHASE 1
Portion Size Reduction and Substitution

Weeks 1 and 2

Over the course of these two weeks, from whichever eating pattern you are starting—omnivore, flexitarian, pescatarian, vegetarian—you will reduce the portion sizes of the Transition Foods by half and add other whole nutritious foods to your meals.

Here are examples for each eating pattern showing how, within any given day, you can reduce your Transition Food portions and make substitutions.

Omnivore > Flexitarian

Since the goal of becoming flexitarian is to reduce your red and processed meat intake, if you typically eat two fried eggs and two pork sausages for breakfast, eat one pork sausage, and substitute the other with a turkey sausage and side of fruit. If you usually have four slices of ham in your ham and cheese sandwich, remove two of the ham slices and add avocado, lettuce, or cucumber (or all of the above) for volume. Instead of six ounces of rib-eye steak with creamed spinach and potatoes au gratin on the side for dinner, eat three ounces of steak with sautéed spinach and roasted potatoes. In each case, you are cutting your red and processed meat consumption in half and substituting it with more nutritious alternatives. This will ensure you are not only making healthier choices but also still feeling full and satisfied.

Flexitarian > Pescatarian

The goal here is to reduce your consumption of white meat and continue cutting down on processed foods. For lunch, instead of topping your salad with six ounces of chicken, top it with three ounces of chicken, and substitute the rest with a legume, cheese, or nuts. For dinner, eat a fish-based appetizer (e.g. shrimp cocktail), so that by the time you get to your main course, in this example turkey chili, it will be easy to cut down six ounces of ground turkey to three ounces, while adding more vegetables and beans to make up for the meat. In this transition, it is important to add additional whole foods that are high in iron, protein, and other vitamins that you may be getting less of while reducing meat intake.

Pescatarian > Vegetarian

In this transition you are reducing your fish consumption, so for lunch, rather than eating a macro bowl with six ounces of salmon, white rice, and broccoli, eat three ounces of salmon with brown rice (always choose whole grains over refined grains when possible), lentils, and broccoli. Similarly, if you have been eating eight ounces of shrimp with zucchini sautéed in butter and a side of cream- and butter-laden mashed potatoes for dinner, cut the shrimp back to four ounces, keep the zucchini but sauté it in olive oil, add a second sauteéd vegetable such as eggplant or asparagus, and replace the cream in the mashed potatoes with plant-based milk, or even a white bean puree, which has more protein and fiber.

Vegetarian > Vegan

Since you are starting out as a vegetarian, you have already cut out all meats and fish, but want to continue cutting down the remaining animal products. If you have been using butter, replace it with vegetable oils (e.g. extra virgin olive, rapeseed, or canola) or plant-based butter. If you have been making smoothies with milk, start making them with half milk and half plant-based milk and add nut butter. If you are used to eating a two-egg omelet with veggies and cheese for breakfast, make your omelet with one egg and half the amount of cheese (you can also add a vegan JUST Egg and vegan cheese for bulk if desired), and add a side of fruit or slice of seed bread to compensate. For lunch, if you are used to eating two slices of cheese in your sandwich, have one, or if you usually toss a quarter cup of feta, goat, or blue cheese on your salad, cut back to an eighth of a cup. As replacements you can begin to substitute the dairy cheese you are reducing with vegan and nut-based cheese and ingredients like nutritional yeast, which has a cheese-like flavor.

By the end of Week 2, you should be eating only half your Transition Foods any time they appear in a meal.

If you're comfortable with this phase, I encourage you to continue to Phase 2. However, if you feel like you need more time to adjust, read the Assessment section that follows (see page 39) and take another week to master this phase.

PHASE 2
Transition Food Frequency Reduction

Weeks 3 and 4

Now that you have reduced the portion sizes of your Transition Foods, weeks three and four are designated for you to work on reducing the number of meals per day that incorporate your Transition Food. If you are still eating the Transition Foods as part of two to three meals per day, for each eating pattern you will focus on reducing your consumption of them to ONE meal per day.

The below examples focus on substituting out transition foods at specific meals but remember, in addition to replacing these foods, which this section highlights, you should be keeping and/or adding vegetables, fruit, whole grains, and other plant-based alternatives to them as well.

Omnivore > Flexitarian

If you have been eating fried eggs and a pork sausage in the morning, a ham and cheese sandwich at lunch, and a hamburger for dinner, replace the red and processed meats in two of your meals with white meat, fish, eggs, dairy, legumes, or other vegetarian alternatives. For example, you could substitute the pork sausage with turkey sausage and the ham with chicken salad, and add some vegetables to your dishes (i.e., celery, pickles, lettuce, and tomato to your chicken salad) or a side of fruit. You could also keep your pork sausage and substitute during lunch and dinner, or keep the ham sandwich and substitute during breakfast and dinner; it does not matter which meals with red and processed meat you eliminate, but if you're eating three of these in a day, you must get rid of two.

Flexitarian > Pescatarian

If you have been eating a turkey bacon omelet in the morning and roast chicken at night as your mains, choose to keep either the turkey bacon in the omelet for breakfast **OR** the chicken for dinner. Replace the bacon with vegetarian bacon or smoked salmon **OR** the chicken with halibut, and make sure to include a side of fruit with your breakfast and healthy vegetable sides with your dinner.

Pescatarian > Vegetarian

If you eat fish twice a day, say a salad with tuna for lunch and cod for dinner, choose either the tuna **OR** the cod. You can replace the tuna with legumes (e.g., chickpeas, lentils, cannellini beans), a hard-boiled egg, or tempeh for instance, **OR** the cod with one of many plant-based protein options like tofu or seitan. Again, round out your meals with a variety of fresh vegetables and fruit sides.

Vegetarian > Vegan

If you have been eating scrambled eggs for breakfast, salad with cheese for lunch, and macaroni and cheese for dinner, pick two meals at which to forgo eggs and dairy. You can substitute the scrambled eggs with a tofu and vegetable scramble **OR** the cheese in your salad with nuts, seeds, and vegan cheese. If the mac and cheese is going to go, the good news is you do not have to eliminate it all together because recipes on the Internet abound for vegan macaroni and cheese. You can also make regular pasta with cashew-cream based sauces.

By the end of weeks three and four, only ONE meal a day should contain your transition food group. If you are comfortable at this point move to Phase 3. If you need more time, read the Assessment section which might convince you to try this phase for another week.

PHASE 3
Days Per Week Reduction

Weeks 5 and 6

Since you are now eating the Transition Food Group only once per day, during weeks five and six, you will turn your attention to reducing the number of days per week on which you eat those foods. In week five you will reduce the number of your Transition Foods days by half (e.g. six days to three days), and in week six you will eliminate the Transition Foods on ALL the remaining days.

The below examples model how you will complete your transition in its entirety from one eating pattern to another.

Omnivore > Flexitarian

If you are moving from omnivore to flexitarian and have succeeded in eating red and processed meat once per day but are still consuming them on four days of the week, replace two meals in which they occur in week five, and then the remaining two meals in week six. For example, in week five, you could swap a Canadian bacon egg sandwich, with a meat-free omelet, and a lunch salad topped with steak, with organic chicken instead. In week six, for the remaining two meals, if you need to swap out a veal Milanese and a pork loin, you could exchange them with a chicken Milanese and pan-fried breaded fillet of fish.

Note: if you do not want to give up red and processed meat altogether as a flexitarian, you do not have to. You can read more about how to incorporate these infrequently on holidays and special occasions in the guide for The Flexitarian (see page 61).

Flexitarian > Pescatarian

In week five, if you are eating white meat four days a week, reduce your consumption of it to two days. For example, you could swap a chicken-based stir fry with a meatless stir fry and chicken tinga tacos with shrimp tacos. In week six, eliminate the last two days on which you eat meat entirely. Eat anchovies on your lunch salad instead of chicken or a fillet of sea bass instead of turkey breast for dinner.

Pescatarian > Vegetarian

To reduce your fish consumption on two days of the week in week five, replace the salmon in your salad with hard-boiled eggs, cheese, legumes, seitan, tofu, or tempeh, and choose tempeh or tofu tacos instead of Baja fish tacos. In week six, eliminate the remaining two days on which you eat fish, substituting them with vegetarian alternatives. Replace a crab cake with a black bean burger, or a tuna salad sandwich with an egg salad sandwich.

Vegetarian > Vegan

If you are still consuming milk, cream, eggs, and cheese on six days of the week in week five, and three days in week six, here are a few ideas for how to swap them out. In week five, trade in your Greek yogurt parfait for a parfait made with coconut-based yogurt. If it's taco night, make a vegetable, tempeh, or seitan taco and begin experimenting with vegan cheese and tofu sour cream. If eggs are your protein staple in salads, replace them with legumes, nuts, seeds, or tofu. In week six, make your overnight oats with almond milk instead of regular milk, your pasta with bolognaise sauce made with one of the many plant-based ground meat options, and your pizza with vegan mozzarella. As you experience being vegan, you will begin to realize that there is a world of vegan-friendly alternatives for almost any of the foods you ate before.

If you were able to complete your transition by the end of week six, you will officially be a flexitarian, pescatarian, vegetarian, or vegan, and it is time for Phase 4. If not, keep reading anyway. You too are on your way!

PHASE 4
Honing and Maintenance

Weeks 7 and 8

If you have successfully adhered to the schedule thus far, I would like you to carry on with the eating pattern established at the end of week six and use these two weeks to let your body and mind adjust to your new diet before moving on to a different eating pattern or deciding that this is the eating pattern for you, for life. Weeks seven and eight are built in to focus solely on maintenance. If you transitioned from being an omnivore to a flexitarian, then maintain your flexitarian status, a flexitarian to pescatarian, then stay pescatarian, and so on and so forth.

As I mentioned at the beginning of this section, however, you might need more time than the allocated eight weeks to complete your transition to a new eating pattern, and if this is the case, do not stress. Whereas two months is comfortable for some, for others, the shift can be too rapid, and there is nothing wrong with that. So next, I will delve into how to assess yourself to decide if you need to decelerate your transition. Remember, the goal is sustainability, not a race against the calendar.

Assessment Exercises

Assessment is the process by which you will track and evaluate how you are doing as you progress between the different lifestyles. Monitoring your progress is crucial to any diet transformation because it allows you to acquire information that can indicate if your plan is working for you.

As you make changes to your diet, it is critical that you take a step back at the end of each week, each two-week period, and at the end of the eight-week period to check in with how you feel in body, mind, and spirit. This requires planning a few minutes each Sunday (or a regular time that is convenient for your schedule) to sit quietly and meditate on how your new eating pattern is affecting you physically, emotionally, and psychologically. Find a quiet place to sit for five minutes. Set a timer and close your eyes. Focus on your breath and turn your awareness inward. Try to get an overall sense of how you're feeling, whether you're restless and anxious, or peaceful and calm. When you're done, grab a journal and do the exercise below.

Journal Exercise

Here are three sets of questions that will help you evaluate where you are with your transitioning. I would like you to do this exercise for all the diets you try. Write your answers in a notebook or journal so that you can always refer to them. Depending on the answers, you might refine your approach.

Set 1: The Experience

- Do I feel adequately nourished with energy to do everything I want to do (family, work, exercise, relationships, friendships, house chores)?
- Am I feeling satiated with my food consumption (full and that the foods I am eating are tasty) or deprived (hungry and like I've given up too many foods I love to eat)? If satiated, explain why in some detail. If

deprived, ask yourself how you could turn your feelings of scarcity into abundance. (Could I make better substitutions? Do I need more time? More variety?)

- What environmental, social, family, and other external influences are impacting me? Are they positive or negative? What are three strategies I can employ to bolster the positive and reduce the negative?
- What was easy for me about this eating pattern, and why?
- What was challenging for me about this eating pattern, and why?

Set 2: Well-Being Check

- Describe how your body feels. Does it feel stronger or weaker? Agile or clumsy? Inflamed or calm? Did you gain weight? Did you lose weight? (I don't particularly advocate using scales; you can if you want but you can also assess your weight by how your clothes fit, how you look, asking a trusted loved one, and by how you feel.)
- Describe your emotions. Have you been feeling stressed, angry, anxious, frustrated, discouraged, ineffective, lacking in self-esteem, unmotivated, irritable, or depressed? On the contrary, have you been feeling in control, confident, productive, excited, happy, at ease, accomplished, or calm? These are just some examples but write your precise feelings.
- Describe your thoughts. Have you been obsessing, ruminating, and absent-minded or clear-minded, focused, and on top of your game? Have you been engaging in catastrophic black-and-white thinking or measured and even keeled?
- If you could change one thing about your experience, what would it be?

Set 3: Medical Check

- Have I met with my dietician and/or physician and is my nutritional status adequate (caloric intake, macro- and micronutrients)?

If most of your answers to these questions are positive and you are nutritionally sound (and your doctor gives you the green light), you can feel confident that the eating pattern with which you are working is promising and could be right for you long term. You can also tackle the next eating pattern if you have the desire.

If most of your answers are negative, try to improve your experience with your current eating pattern and wait before moving on. Spend some more time evaluating why the current plan has not been working for you. Is the schedule too compressed and could the eating pattern be successful if you extended it? Do you need to personalize your modifications of portion sizes, meal frequency, and days to a greater degree? Do you love the foods you are eliminating so much you just do not feel you want to remove them completely? Do you need to take cooking lessons to learn how to better prepare the foods in the new plan? Do you need more support from your family, friends, and community, or medical, nutritional, and psychotherapeutic professionals? Are you having any unusual physiological problems or symptoms? (If so, visit your nutritionist or doctor.) Is the diet perhaps just not right for you? Be honest with yourself. The last thing I want is for you to land in a framework that feels forced, uncomfortable, or is counterproductive to achieving your goals.

How to Navigate
Eating Anywhere

Aspects of the environments in which we eat often pose the biggest challenges to a successful shift in diet because the external forces of work schedules, family commitments, and social life can make nutrition goals feel impossible to achieve. But it doesn't have to be this way. Here are a few tips that will help you conquer some potential pitfalls. We will delve deeper into many aspects of these within the specific eating patterns in the chapters to come.

Cooking at Home

The more you can cook at home the better. Shoot for at least five homemade breakfasts, lunches, and dinners per week. Working in an office can make this more challenging, but with focused planning, you can prepare meals at home and bring them with you to work when convenient.

Refurbish your kitchen to suit your new lifestyle. Get rid of foods you don't want to be eating any longer and stock up with the ingredients you need to prepare the dishes in your new meal plan. Try organizing your space in a way that makes cooking easy and quick, cleaning efficient, and maintenance possible. For instance, invest in a line of matching pantry jars in different sizes so you can easily access your ingredients and get rid of clunky, messy packaging. Separate your fruits and vegetables in different refrigerator drawers according to how and when you most commonly use them. Keep all your consistently used condiments together. Organize your machines and utensils in the most easily accessible drawers and according to how frequently you use them. And remember to clean as you cook, replacing things where they belong so as not to let disorder set in once again.

Find a convenient and efficient system for food shopping that works for you on a regular basis. Are you going to go to the stores on the weekend, going on your days off, or ordering groceries online? Will you always be the shopper or is there another family member or someone who works for you who can assist you? Do you have time for meal preparation each day or do you need to allot a few hours each week to chop vegetables for salads, make soups you can freeze, soak your legumes, and prepare your grains?

Buy shelf-stable ingredients you will use on a regular basis like spices, condiments, whole grains, legumes, nuts, seeds, and baking components.

Make sure you have the equipment you will need to execute your recipes. One way to do this is by going through some recipes you plan to cook and see if they call for any tools that you don't already own. Social media and cooking websites are also great places to learn about kitchen essentials. It's more likely you'll cook these recipes if you are prepared.

Meal plans make life easier because they reduce the amount of time and thought put toward food in any given hectic workday, so write yours in advance of the week ahead. If any unforeseen events crop up during the week, your meal plan serves as an adaptable foundation off which you can work. Also use this time to select recipes for the week (read more about meal planning on page 116).

Eating at the Office

When you can, bring your lunch from home. This enables you to exert full control over what you will consume while eliminating the stress of what, where, when, and how you will procure the appropriate foods for your plan. Avoid produce such as avocado and sliced apples (whole ones are great), which go bad quickly and don't travel well.

If your office does not have a communal refrigerator, consider getting your own mini fridge to keep by your desk so that your healthy foods stay fresh (salads and fruit, some of the things I encourage you to eat for lunch or a snack, do best when kept cool).

If you cannot bring your lunch to work, pick two or three places close by to which you can go or from which you can order in, and let these be your go-to haunts. Make sure each has at least a couple of options that appeal to you and that the portion sizes served are appropriate (portion size when buying work lunches is one of the biggest pitfalls, so really take your time on this). It is ideal if the foods available at the establishments you choose are fresh, whole, and organic.

Avoid company treats and foods that are left out (like candy bowls), circulated (caloric coffee drinks), or presented for celebrations (yes, kindly decline those cupcakes). They are generally unhealthy and should not be in your plan unless it's a truly special occasion and you adjust your meal plan to account for them.

If you must attend a company meeting with a meal in the office, try to participate in the planning and ordering process (at least give word to the person who is doing the ordering about what your requirements are) or choose the healthiest option available within the parameters of your eating pattern. However, don't be shy about bringing something you made from home. Today, people are generally understanding about various nutrition needs and your health is more important than others' opinions of you.

Dining Out

Avoid eating out as much as possible (shoot for less than twice a week for any meal). Given work schedules, you might have less control, but do your best to limit those dining-out work obligations.

Sticking with appetizers is a great way to manage portion control. That said, be cautious if you are at the kind of restaurant where one appetizer could feed an entire family! If this is the case, try to share or only eat as much as is appropriate.

If you would still like to order a main course dish, again consider portion size, which can be enormous at restaurants. Do not be afraid to ask your server before ordering about how much food is in a certain dish. Once you have this essential information, you can decide:

- If you want to order the dish all to yourself knowing you'll need to implement the discipline to eat half or less (take the rest home if you would like).
- If you want to ask if it's possible to order a smaller portion (for instance half an order or the smallest cut of meat or fish they have).
- If you want to share it with someone else at the table.
- If you want to order something completely different instead.

Knowing the ingredients with which dishes are prepared—especially if you are vegetarian or vegan, have an allergy, or are trying to watch your weight—is even more crucial for those who want to be strict about their diet. Again, do not be afraid to ask! Many restaurants are willing to accommodate personal preferences and if they are not, you'll know where to avoid. (If eating out is an infrequent occurrence, you can also consider being more relaxed about your diet on these rare occasions.) If you cannot find anything you want on the main menu, try making a meal out of a few sides.

Alcohol in moderation is okay. The 2020–2025 USDA recommendations suggest that the less you drink, the better, but if you are going to drink, it's best to consume no more than one glass a day for women and no more than two glasses a day for men. I, however, believe in being more stringent about my alcohol intake and choose one night a week on which to drink it, usually between Thursday and Saturday, the days on which I most likely go out with friends. On vacations and holidays, I'm happy to give a little on this.

Delivery/Takeout

Avoid takeout and delivery as much as possible. Unlike in restaurants, it's much more difficult to get accurate answers and make swaps and customizations when taking food out from a restaurant than it is when dining in one. Rather than go down that road, have on hand some quick and easy options you can throw together at home, like whole wheat or Banza pasta and tomato sauce, or homemade meals and leftovers you've frozen like vegetarian burgers, soups, or chicken skewers you prepared the previous weekend that just require being heated up.

On the occasions when you must order food in or do take out, get to know the places around you that serve the healthiest options and suitable portions. Read menus and reviews online, call to ask questions in advance, and ask a neighbor or a friend who has been to verify what you've discovered.

Be aware of your eyes being bigger than your stomach. It's easy and common to get overly excited by a menu, especially when you're hungry, and end up ordering too much food. The consequences? Overeating, throwing out perfectly good food (reducing food waste is definitely important to include in your plant-based goal set), and feeling guilty. It's best to start by ordering less because you can always top off lingering hunger with something healthy from your kitchen.

Finding a Supportive Community

With whom we surround ourselves has a large impact on our consumption habits and behaviors, so pick your eating companions carefully. For many, this starts at home. The more knowledge those around you have about your goals and the reasons behind them, the more helpful and encouraging they can be. You can ask your family, significant other, and roommates to try a new eating pattern with you for fun or to keep tempting processed foods out of sight, if not out of the house entirely. If you are making a new recipe, see if they would like to join and cook with you, or at least share the finished product. If you are watching a documentary on the environment, animal rights, or healthy eating, invite them to watch with you. The value-add of this welcoming approach is that everyone gets the opportunity to reap the rewards—they too might lose some weight, improve their overall health status, find a new dish they love, or develop a greater consciousness about climate change and animal welfare. Everyone can win!

But while you can ask for support from family, romantic partners, and roommates, you cannot expect that they will be as excited as you and jump on your bandwagon. They might, in fact, have a disappointing reaction to your new lifestyle. If this is the case, try to find other like-minded people outside of the home who get it. You could:

- Join an online or social media community that supports what you are doing.
- Enroll in a book club whose defining component is wellness.
- Participate in a walking, running, cycling, or tennis group, or make friends at your gym (people who get together for group exercise tend to be more mindful about diet).

- Sign up for a cooking class or a course on nutrition.
- Hire a coach or therapist with whom you can work.

You are bound to encounter people who are not on your page, but the key is not to let them stymie you. Trust your internal compass and embolden your conviction by surrounding yourself with people who are supportive, aligned, positive, and motivated.

Embracing Exercise

Exercise is a necessary component of any healthy lifestyle regardless of your eating pattern. Since 2008, the Department of Health and Human Services has put forth Physical Activity Guidelines for Americans, which calls for at least 150 to 300 minutes of moderate aerobic exercise or 75 to 150 minutes of vigorous exercise spread throughout the week. In addition, the guidelines recommend at least two days a week of strength-training, whether with weights and machines or your own body weight. The purpose of the guidelines is to help people understand how much and what type of activity is required to reap important health benefits. Carve out some time daily, even if it's just ten-minute bouts three times a day on busy days, to devote to your fitness regimen.

If you are thinking this means you have to start training for a triathlon, this is absolutely not the case. Most movement counts as physical activity, from house chores like vacuuming and gardening; to recreational exercise like walking, jogging, and yoga; to sports like swimming and playing basketball. Even just playing around in the yard with your kids counts.

Science journals publish new evidence daily about the benefits of exercise on all different aspects of our health and wellbeing. For example, new research highlights the benefits of fitness on:

- Diabetes
- Cardiovascular health
- Cancer
- Obesity
- High blood pressure
- Brain health
- Bone health
- Auto-immune disease
- Muscle strength and health
- Fall-related injuries
- Mood and psychological disorders
- Aging

This is a short list, which could certainly go on. The point is, in addition to having a healthy nutrition plan, spending less time being sedentary and more time being active is equally important to achieving truly meaningful wellness results, no matter your age. I have worked with many clients upwards of seventy years old who are strong, mobile, clear-minded, and living it up. They attribute their well-being to their consistent fitness efforts throughout life, especially in the later years, even if at that point their activities are less aggressive. Walking, yoga, Pilates, tennis, biking, gardening, and swimming are a few physical activities that aren't too hard on the body and have an amazing effect as age sets in.

To feel your best, ensure your body will be in balance, and avoid overuse injuries, I recommend alternating days on which you do cardio and strength/flexibility training. For instance, you could do aerobic activity on Monday, Wednesday, Friday, and Sunday, and strength and flexibility on Tuesday and Thursday, with Saturday as a rest day. If you are extremely active or an athlete, at least one rest day—if not two—a week, is necessary to let your body rest, repair, and recover.

Practicing Mindfulness

Any plant-based lifestyle will benefit from mindfulness. Mindfulness is the act of being in the moment. You would be surprised to know how much time the average mind of a human being spends in the past and future as opposed to the present. We ruminate about a work project gone awry the prior day or week or worry about whether we can make our romantic relationship last into the future. We stress about a poor grade our child got on a test in school or we get anxious about the to-do list we have for the week ahead.

There is no better arena than nutrition to hone our mindfulness skills. The idea of going plant-based is an inherently mindful decision because it demands that you observe how you can best serve yourself, the planet, and animals. Moreover, it is not about creating change in a year or five years. It is about getting started now and showing up for yourself every day with a deliberate approach toward that which you put in your body.

Mindful eating, also known as intuitive eating, calls for being conscious not only about what you eat, but also about how you consume your food. Regardless of the eating pattern, the more mindful you can be as you progress, the more success you will have. There are many facets of mindful eating, which studies show results in lower calorie intake, but here is a list of a few I would like you to practice as you start your new plant-based life:

- Listen to your internal hunger and satiety cues. If you're full, stop eating. If you're hungry, eat more. This might seem obvious, but most people do not adhere to this principle and just eat for the sake of eating because the food is in front of them, they're watching TV, others around are doing so, or because it's convenient. Also remember that it takes your brain twenty minutes to register fullness, so if you've eaten enough but still have an edge of hunger, wait. The Hunger-Satiety Scale (also known as The Hunger-Fullness Scale), which is a visual analog scale often used in nutritional research, is a great tool you can use to assess your level of hunger and satiation with ratings from one to ten. (The idea is to determine when you are comfortably satisfied and neither hungry nor over-full.)

- Eat slowly, chewing your food at least twenty times, making eating an experience—rather than a rush, which can lead to excess intake.

- Engage your senses by smelling your food, seeing the colors of it, noticing its presentation, and acknowledging its texture—from hearing the sounds of the preparation to its mouthfeel (e.g. Crunchy? Smooth? Cool? Hot? Chewy? Soft? Tough?)

- Plate your food on appropriately sized plates with equally appropriate portion sizes. Several studies have shown that when the same portion of food is presented on a small versus a large plate, we can be more satisfied with the food on the small plate even though it is the same amount. The mind plays tricks on us making us think that the large plate has less food on it because our eyes see more empty space, which registers as scarcity and feeling less satisfied (this is known as the Delbouf Illusion). While not all studies support usage of small plates to achieve portion control, I've found that the technique works for me and my clients.

- Be device-free at mealtimes. Many studies show that eating when distracted on smartphones, computers, or while watching television can increase calorie intake.

- Engage in social conversation at the table. Maintaining strong and positive social connections with family and friends, which is often accomplished at mealtimes, has shown to enhance health and longevity.

- Pay attention to meal timing. Eat your meals (two or three of them) at approximately the same time every day with three- to four-hour breaks in between. (Have one small healthy afternoon snack if truly necessary.) Both eating breakfast in the morning and intermittent fasting (having your first meal—breakfast—in the late morning) show evidence of success with weight loss and chronic disease prevention. The key is to eat consistently within a twelve-hour time frame every day, however, NOT within two hours of bedtime, which is associated with weight gain and decreased glucose tolerance. Following these protocols sets our biological clock and metabolism up for the greatest success while also helping to curb nutrient-poor cravings.

- Create a calming, attractive environment in which you enjoy your food. Warm colors, candles, nice tablecloths, flowers, music, and meaningful objects can all reduce stress during the dining experience, which facilitates intuitive food intake.

- If you are susceptible to emotional eating, take out a pen and journal and answer the following questions: 1) What is making me feel upset, anxious, or stressed? 2) Have I been depriving myself of certain foods lately (this could be why I'm making excuses to eat emotionally)? 3) What methods other than eating can I use to soothe my emotions (e.g. Exercise? Chat with a friend? Play a board game? Read? Get crafty? Meditate? Nap? Play with my dog?)?

Nurturing Yourself

Establishing any new nutrition habit, behavior, or routine requires discipline, patience, perseverance, and self-love. Creating a life change is not always fun. You will be frustrated at times. You will think you are a failure. You will mess up and want to give into cravings. You will get tired and even down. When this happens, be compassionate toward yourself. Corral your cheerleaders and talk to them about your feelings. Reflect so that you can figure out what is working, what is driving the challenges facing you, and how you can conquer them. And remind yourself that every day is a new day, which means you can restart and refresh every morning. (I am a big believer that breakfast is indeed the most important meal of the day for many reasons including the fact that it is a daily opportunity to reset.)

When things are tough, here are a few ways you can be kind to yourself. Attend a weekend wellness or yoga retreat, walk or hike in nature, or sit by a body of water. There are few things in life more cathartic and life affirming than immersing yourself in nature and exercising. That said, for those of you who are in an urban environment like I often am: take a stroll through a museum or by the river; see a live theatrical show; go to the city's botanical garden, parks, or zoo; take a bike ride; or call up a friend for a drink or dinner. Get a massage. Get your nails done. Get lost in a book or an iconic movie. Line up your resources so that you can easily take a train or drive to the countryside or beach. Do things that genuinely make you happy and grounded, that reconnect you with the essence of life and vitality, and that take your mind off the incredibly difficult—albeit most rewarding—thing you are doing for yourself: finding the fuel that best charges you and your life.

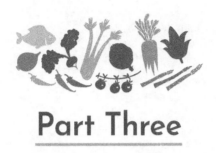

Part Three

THE DIETS

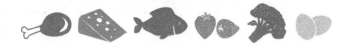

Diet 1: The Flexitarian

The term flexitarian combines two concepts: flexible and vegetarian. The flexitarian diet refers to an eating pattern that is mostly vegetarian, but includes moderate amounts of animal-sourced products. In 2003, the American Dialect Society recognized "flexitarian" as one of the most important emerging words in the English language, though its use was limited primarily to the foodie and culinary communities. It wasn't until around 2009 that the flexitarian eating pattern gained broader appeal for a rapidly growing segment of the population: people who want to eat vegetarian much of the time in order to reap the health benefits of this diet, but who also want to continue eating some meat, fish, dairy, and eggs. Unlike most diets, the flexitarian diet is not all-or-nothing, but tips the balance toward a plant-based life.

Given that a flexitarian diet allows for all forms of animal-sourced products, why does it qualify as plant-based? The reason many dieticians, nutritionists, academics, and other health experts consider this eating pattern to be plant-based is because it promotes increased consumption of plant foods (fruits, vegetables, whole grains, nuts, seeds, legumes, and vegetarian proteins) and decreased consumption of meat (especially red and processed), pork, and poultry. Think of it this way: most flexitarians eat four or more meatless meals a week, in contrast to omnivores who may eat few, if any, meatless meals per week.

Because it is a relatively unrestrictive way to improve diet quality, the flexitarian approach appeals to many, including those who plan to stay flexitarian and those who seek to use it as a stepping stone for the other plant-based diets covered in this guide. If you are an omnivore with the goal of becoming pescatarian, vegetarian, or vegan, I highly recommend starting here. Incrementally removing animal-sourced products from your diet will give you the opportunity to assess how you feel at various stages, as your body and mind adjust to gradual shifts in food choices. It will also increase the likelihood that you will be able to maintain your new healthy eating pattern for the long term.

Evidence is clear about what doesn't work: drastic diet changes that shock the body and make us feel deprived, sending hunger and cravings through the roof. A flexitarian diet is the opposite: a big-tent approach that allows for a lot of experimentation and customization within the realm of plant-based eating.

In this chapter, I will provide you with some cherry-picked guidelines for understanding and implementing a flexitarian diet, which I have seen my clients follow with great success. You will learn how to reduce your consumption of meat, enhance the quality of animal-sourced products you eat, and maintain variety in your diet so you never feel deprived.

How to Become Flexitarian: Steps and Implementation

1. **Do the math and reduce your meat intake.** On the flexitarian diet, your goal is not to eliminate meat from your diet altogether, but to eat less of it. For the average adult on a 2,000 calorie diet, the USDA guidelines recommend a maximum of twenty-six ounces of meat, poultry, and eggs per week, and five to six ounces on average per day from the protein group as a whole (thirty-five to forty-two ounces for the average person per week), which, in addition to meat, poultry, and eggs, also includes fish, nuts, seeds, legumes, and other vegetarian proteins such as tofu and tempeh. It's important to eat a variety of all these foods while considering the key things we know about them. As mentioned in Part One, meat is the least healthy of the group. Fish is considered very healthy and the USDA, along with numerous studies, recommends eating at least eight ounces of it per week for its heart-healthy benefits. According to many studies, it's safe to consume up to seven eggs per week without increasing your risk of all-cause mortality (unless you have diabetes or are at risk of heart disease, in which case you should keep it to three or fewer eggs per week). Legumes (including soybeans and derivative products), nuts, and seeds are some of the most nutrient-dense foods on the planet and evidence shows they reduce all-cause mortality.

   Implementation: Consider what you typically eat from the protein group, then compare how this stacks up to USDA guidelines, focusing on meat and poultry consumption. Then reassess and redesign your meal plan in accordance with both the guidelines and your personal goals.

- Get out a notepad and calculator and ask yourself the following question: Will I be eating fish, eggs, nuts, seeds, beans, and other plant-based proteins, and if so, how much of each? Say you answer yes to all these foods because you want maximum variety. Then start to assign values to the quantities of the protein types you plan to eat. For example, if in a week you're going to eat eight ounces of fish, four eggs (one egg is the equivalent of one ounce), twelve ounces of nuts and seeds (one ounce of nuts equals two ounces of protein), five ounces of legumes (a fourth of a cup is the equivalent of one protein ounce), and six ounces of other plant-based proteins like tofu or tempeh, you can begin to see that there's very little room, if any, left for meat, unless you cut down on the other subgroups, which as we know, are healthier. In this example, we're up to thirty-five ounces of protein for the week when the range for the whole group (based on five to six-and-a-half ounces per day) should be between thirty-five on the low end for less active people and forty-six ounces on the high end for very active people. So, the big question is, where and how can you fit meat and poultry in? The answer is very infrequently and in small amounts. Now, I'm not saying you must strictly adhere to the guidelines; your individual needs always come first, and you might need or choose to eat more of one food type than another or change it up week-to-week. I'm just saying, be conscious of what, how much, and why you're making your choices, especially with regards to the meat and poultry you're consuming (the less meat you consume, the better).

- Next, take back control of how much meat and poultry you're actually eating. Here's how: ask your butcher for a specific number of ounces of meat instead of a quantity for a certain number of people (with a non-specific direction, you can be sure that you will get far more than you want). At home, check to see that your portions approximate the size of a deck of cards, and if they don't, cut them down (a standard card deck is a good visual representation of what approximately three ounces of meat looks like). Invest in a food scale, which is a relatively inexpensive one-time purchase, and weigh your meat on your own. When eating out, ask the server how many ounces of meat will be served in your dish, and if it is more than you would like, eat half and take home the rest, share with a dinner companion, or order an appetizer or something else instead. People who subscribe to the flexitarian eating pattern range vastly in their meat consumption; how much meat you eat is entirely up to you, but eating less can have the triple benefit of improving your health, the environment, and animal welfare.

2. **Avoid processed meats.** Flexitarianism can seem complicated because so many foods are fair game when consumed in moderation. With this step, I am going to make things simple for you by asking you to eschew the unhealthiest types of meat all together: those that are highly processed. Meat in fast food hamburgers, tacos, and hot dogs, for instance, is loaded with artery-clogging, heart-harming saturated fat, cholesterol, sodium, hormones, antibiotics, chemicals, and other unnatural ingredients, which damage the human body. The same goes for deli meats, which, in addition to containing similar disease-causing components, also contain nitrates and nitrites. Nitrates and nitrites are chemicals used mostly in cured meats like salami, sausage, bacon, and roast beef, to give them the pinkish red color that appeals to our eyes, but also can be carcinogenic. Finally, processed meat is produced on factory farms, which as you now know, are incredibly harmful to the environment and animals.

   Implementation: If you feel that you can't avoid processed meat all together, rather than heading to your favorite fast-food haunts, at least upgrade to higher quality fast casual destinations. Beef at some fast casual chains like Chipotle and Panera gets A and A- ratings respectively on the annual Chain Reaction Antibiotics scorecard (an annual report that grades America's top restaurant chains on their policies and methods regarding their antibiotic use and candidness in their meat and poultry supply chains), whereas beef from the most popular fast food franchises gets ratings that range from C to F. If convenience and affordability remain obstacles to making this upgrade, most fast food chains now provide vegetarian options, which would be your next best choice.

3. **Substitute red meat with white meat, fish, and vegetarian proteins.** White meat, fish, and vegetarian proteins are lower in saturated fat and sodium and higher in polyunsaturated fats and omega-3s than red meat. Red meat dishes are also frequently served with sides such

as french fries, onion rings, and creamed spinach, which are also rich in saturated fats. Now that you know how much meat you want to include in your diet and are making a shift away from processed meat, it's time to start swapping as much red meat out of your meal plan as possible.

Implementation: Healthy mornings set the tone for the rest of the day and breakfast is, for many, the easiest meal to modify. Most red breakfast meats have white-meat or vegetarian alternatives, so if those foods are part of your morning routine, try swapping bacon for its turkey counterpart or regular sausage for vegetarian sausage. What's more, many popular healthy breakfast options such as oatmeal, eggs, and smoothies are naturally vegetarian. Once you have breakfast down, apply the same approach to lunch. If your regular weekday lunch is a salami sandwich, substitute the salami with turkey or Tofurky. Once you have started to enjoy the benefits of reducing your red meat intake during the day, consider making similar swaps at dinner. Rather than steak frites, creamed spinach, and french fries, have roast chicken or a piece of grilled fish with sautéed kale and a baked sweet potato on the side. Your gut will thank you, because eating healthy in the evenings reduces the amount of digestive work, which in turn can yield a deeper and higher-quality sleep.

4. **Save your red meat for special occasions.** Reserving your red meat consumption for special occasions is another easy way to curb your intake. Holidays, birthdays, graduations, weddings, and other celebratory gatherings warrant a more laissez-faire attitude than an average Friday night and should be times when you can ease up on your rulebook.

Implementation: Get out a calendar and mark the most important upcoming celebrations. Be particular about which times are truly most meaningful to you, because otherwise, you will very quickly fill up the calendar. Do not include work-related breakfasts, lunches, and dinners, events, or routine meals out with friends. These should be infrequent significant events—family or close friends' birthdays, annual celebrations like Thanksgiving and the Fourth of July, religious holidays, weddings, and graduations. Then, plan to treat yourself on those days to filet mignon or a pork chop.

5. **Educate yourself about animal food production, healthy recipes, and nutrition.** New habits are much more likely to stick when you are informed and passionate about why you are instituting them. As mentioned in Part One, a growing body of information about nutrition and cooking is easily accessible in documentary films (*Biggest Little Farm, What the Health*), carefully selected social media accounts (*drmarkhyman, Nutrition Stripped*), magazines (*Eating Well*), books (*Food Rules, Flavor, The Blue Zones Kitchen*), and scientific journals (*The American Journal of Clinical Nutrition*). The more knowledge you have, the more confident you will be in decisions concerning shopping, cooking, and meal planning for a long-term high-quality diet.

   Implementation: Dedicate some time to learning about animal food production and flexitarian cooking through documentaries, social media, books, and articles such as the ones mentioned in Part One and this step. Then, spend some time searching hashtags and websites that pertain to your new interest in plant-based food and follow relevant social media accounts. To help make the shift in food prep interesting and manageable, start keeping a list of links to recipes that appeal to you or print them and make a book to keep on hand in your kitchen (I like to print and organize my favorites in a binder). A few online resources I recommend for healthy flexitarian recipes include *New York Times Cooking, Epicurious, Bon Appetit, Food and Wine,* and *Food52.* Finally, when you're feeling extra ambitious, search Google and Google Scholar to find evidence-based studies on plant-based nutrition topics that are of particular interest to you. I know this might sound academic and arduous but it is a practical, immediate, and helpful way to get to the bottom of all the food myths circulating in popular culture.

6. **Prepare and cook your meat to reduce its potentially harmful effects.** As you become flexitarian, you'll want to pay attention to how you prepare and cook your meat, because different methods can increase or decrease saturated fat and cancer-causing elements. Red meat is often cooked with ultra-high heat, which increases its cancer-causing potential because the high temperature causes the muscle—due to its protein content—to mutate and create carcinogenic chemicals called heterocyclic amines (HCAs). Moreover, when grilling, fat from fatty cuts of meat drips

into the flames. The flames then convert the fat into another carcinogenic chemical called polyaromatic hydrocarbons (PAHs). As the flames flare up, these PAHs coat the food. Vegetables and fruit on the other hand are protein and fat-free and therefore escape such problems.

Implementation: Buy lean cuts of red meat labeled "sirloin" and "round," and select higher grades such as "choice" or "select" rather than "prime." When purchasing hamburger meat, choose 95 percent extra-lean patties if you can, but if you cannot find those, be sure to remove as much fat as possible prior to cooking and pour excess oil off the patties after cooking. Then choose lower-heat cooking techniques such as baking, roasting, broiling, or stir-frying rather than grilling or deep frying. For white meat like turkey and chicken, make skinless dishes and also choose 90 to 95 percent lean varieties. Finally, if you like game meats, go for them—they're often lower in fat than animals raised for the market.

7. **Purchase the highest-quality animal-derived products you can afford.** Now that you have the knowledge, it's time to put it to use. Although in many other areas of life where more expensive does not necessarily mean better, in this case, that argument holds: the cheapest animal-sourced foods are usually the most detrimental to overall health and the environment, while more expensive choices reflect the quality of the circumstances in which the animal was raised. If you are worried about affordability, consider your savings from your overall reduction of meat, dairy, and eggs. (Most plant-based proteins like legumes, tofu, and tempeh are cheaper than meat and as your health improves, you will save money on healthcare costs). Here is some information that will help you decide what type of meat, eggs, and dairy you will consume from here on in.

Implementation: When you eat meat, eggs, and dairy, choose pasture-raised, grass-fed, and organic varieties from local farms as often as you can. If possible, start shopping at smaller specialty grocers and farmers' markets. While some regular grocery stores sell organic products, most of their products are conventionally raised.

WHAT DO THOSE LABELS MEAN? THE TERMINOLOGY OF MEAT, EGGS, POULTRY, AND DAIRY

MEAT

Farm-Raised Meat: This is meat from animals raised on massive industrial farms. The cows and pigs are kept in confined and generally filthy spaces, often treated with violence, and primarily fed corn or grains. They are regularly injected with large amounts of antibiotics and the cows also with growth hormones. (It's against federal regulations to inject pigs with hormones.)

Organic Meat: To be deemed organic, USDA regulations require that animals are raised in living conditions that accommodate their natural behaviors (like the ability to graze on pastures), fed 100 percent organic feed and forage, and administered neither antibiotics nor hormones.

Pasture-Raised Meat: Meat from animals raised outside on open pastures. These animals can be grass- or grain-fed, or both.

Grass-Fed Meat: Meat from animals that are fed grass and forage plants (i.e., hay) only and neither grain, corn, nor soy. These animals are usually raised on pastures but can also be raised indoors.

EGGS

Farm-Raised aka Caged Eggs: Eggs from hens that are confined to sixty-seven-square-inch spaces each. These hens never see daylight and are fed a diet of soy and corn. Over 90 percent of eggs sold in the United States are from caged hens.

Cage-Free Eggs: Eggs from birds that are uncaged and kept at a distance from others of one square foot, but remain inside barns some or all of the time. They must be able to perch and dust-bathe. Suppliers must follow regulations for stocking density, perching numbers, and nesting boxes. They eat corn and soy feed.

Organic Eggs: To qualify as organic, eggs must come from chickens that inhabit cage-free environments and have access to the outdoors, even if their outdoor area is just a small pen or enclosed yard area. These eggs must also be free of animal byproducts, synthetic fertilizers, pesticides, antibiotics, and hormones, and cannot be fed genetically modified foods. Only natural molting (when birds shed their feathers to make room for new ones as opposed to picking them off each other) is allowed to occur for hens to produce organic eggs.

Pasture-Raised Eggs: Eggs produced from pasture-raised chickens. "Pasture-raised" is not a government regulated term, which means anyone can use it for marketing their product. There are, however, certification organizations that have developed standards. Certified Humane® for example, defines pasture-raised chickens as those who have at least six hours of time outdoors and 108 square feet of pasture. Your best bet for the highest quality pasture-raised eggs is to buy them from local farms that give their chickens plenty of space to roam (no less than 2.5 acres per 1,000 birds) and that raise them organically on living vegetation, which is rotated regularly.

POULTRY

Free-Range Chicken: Chicken from birds that must have access to pastures at least six hours a day. Each hen must have at least two square feet (just shy of 300 square inches) of outdoor space, but this space is not required to have any living vegetation.

Pasture-Raised Chicken: Chicken from birds that must be allowed on at least 108 square feet of pasture (per chicken) for at least six hours each. The pasture must be mainly covered with living vegetation.

DAIRY

Conventional Milk: Made from cows on industrial farms such as those described for farm-raised meat.

Organic Milk: All cows that produce organic milk must be raised unconfined on land that meets organic standards for at least three years prior to harvesting of the crop. These cows must be given 100 percent organic feed. Farmers cannot administer antibiotics, hormones of any kind, pesticide, or any other synthetic chemicals to these animals.

Grass-Fed Milk: Milk that comes from cows that are only fed grass. No corn, other grains, or soy, ever.

8. **Pay attention to overnutrition and misappropriated nutrition rather than undernutrition.** As evidenced by the obesity/overweight epidemic, the American diet is excessive in calories and nutrient-poor food. Although more than half the population meets or exceeds protein and grain food recommendations, even when they meet the USDA guidelines for nutrients and the top-level food groups, they often misappropriate the subgroups. For example, regarding protein consumption, males between fourteen and fifty-one eat well above the meat, poultry, and egg recommendations, while both males and females eat well below the seafood recommendations even though seafood is almost always the healthier choice. As for carbohydrates and grains, refined grain intake is far above the recommendations, whereas whole grain intake is well below them. Finally, most Americans exceed the recommendations for added sugars, saturated fats, and sodium, and under-consume fruits and vegetables, the food groups most essential for health and well-being because they are low in sugar, fat, and sodium, and high in vitamins, minerals, fiber, and antioxidants.

Implementation: As a flexitarian, make it a goal to hit but not exceed your macronutrient targets (on a 2,000 calorie diet—protein: fifty-six grams per day for the average male and forty-six grams per day for the average female; carbs: 225 to 325 grams per day for the average adult; fat: forty-four to seventy-seven grams per day for the average adult) with the most nutrient-dense foods possible such as fruits, vegetables, whole grains, nuts, seeds, legumes, vegetable oils, plant-based proteins, and fish. Simultaneously, start reducing your consumption of foods such as meat, doughnuts, muffins, sandwiches, white pasta, pizza, soda, fruit juice, desserts, and candy because they are the main culprits for overnutrition. Each of these foods can be substituted with healthier alternatives. For instance, eat salads instead of sandwiches and whole wheat or chickpea flour pasta instead of regular (which is made with highly processed refined white flour); try whole wheat, spelt, almond flour, chickpea, or cauliflower-crust pizza; and experiment with low or no-sugar plant-based ice creams. Choose whole grain and sourdough bread over white bread. Even baked goods, such as sweet breads, muffins, loaf cakes, and cookies can be made healthfully with organic unprocessed nutrient-rich ingredients—there are plenty of ideas to get you started in the recipe section of this book.

Is the Flexitarian Eating Pattern Right for You?

The flexitarian eating pattern could be perfect for you if you check the first box below, plus any other box on the list:

☐ You've consulted with your doctor and dietician and are sure it is healthy for you.

☐ You seek health benefits from reducing your animal product consumption. (See pages 6–7 for a list of health conditions that a plant-based diet can improve and information on the association between meat and disease prevention.)

☐ You want to increase your intake of whole, unprocessed plant foods, including fruits, vegetables, whole grains, nuts, seeds, and legumes, and would like to try experimenting with plant-based proteins like tofu, tempeh, seitan, pea protein-based meats (i.e., Beyond or Impossible), and natto.

☐ You love meat, eggs, and dairy and don't want to give any of them up entirely.

☐ You are concerned about climate change and sustainability and want to help preserve the planet.

☐ You are an animal-lover who believes that humans are meant to eat meat, eggs, and dairy, but prefer kinder and more compassionate means of production that transition them from farm-to-table and are kind to the environment.

☐ You've tried eliminating meat from your diet, and for any reason, health-related or not, it didn't work for you.

☐ You are interested in eating out often.

☐ You would like to eliminate certain types of meat for religious reasons.

☐ You are potentially interested in stricter forms of plant-based eating (such as those covered in the following sections of this guide) but want a simple place to start before going more extreme.

If you've said yes to the first box and at least one other, congrats! You're ready to get started. If your doctor has advised you against this diet, then wait until you get the green light.

Trivia

Q: Is pork considered red or white meat?

A: Pork is considered red meat because it contains more myoglobin (a heme iron containing protein that holds oxygen in muscles) than poultry or fish. Meat is categorized as red or white according to the concentration of myoglobin in the animal's muscles, and pork has enough myoglobin to place it in the red meat category.

Q: Why is white meat considered healthier than red?

A: White meat contains significantly less saturated fat than red meat. Saturated fat raises cholesterol, clogs arteries, and increases the risk of heart disease. Furthermore, white meat contains less heme iron, nitrates, and nitrites, as well as other potentially cell-damaging components that can increase the risk of cancer, diabetes, and all-cause mortality when eaten in excess.

Q: Do egg whites count when calculating how many eggs per week to eat?

A: No. Eggs whites are pure, low-fat protein (only thirteen calories per egg white), and unlike egg yolks, they are cholesterol- and saturated fat-free. Although it is not recommended to eat more than seven eggs per week, you need not worry as much about how many egg whites you consume, of course, keeping in mind, everything in moderation. In fact, egg whites are a great way to increase your portion sizes while keeping your consumption of whole eggs to less than seven per week (for instance you can make an omelet with one whole egg and three egg whites).

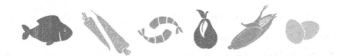

Diet 2: The Pescatarian

I f you're still with me, I am guessing you've had some success reducing your animal product consumption as a flexitarian and are ready to replace the remaining meat in your diet with fish. Welcome to my world: I started my own plant-based journey when I went from omnivore to vegetarian as a teenager, but I turned pescatarian in early adulthood, where I've happily remained ever since.

I was initially inspired to give up eating meat after watching a film on factory farming in high school. I remained vegetarian through college, until, soon after graduating, I started to feel like something was off: my meals seemed monotonous and my body deprived of nutrients. I knew that some people thrived on a vegetarian diet, but it appeared that vegetarianism was no longer a good fit for me. So, in my early twenties, I became a pescatarian and everything changed. With the inclusion of fish and seafood in my eating plan, I felt satiated and excited to eat again. Another perk was that I could go to any restaurant and not feel like a drag for asking the chef to make substitutions every time. (Thankfully the world has changed, and restaurants are *much* more accommodating to patrons with a wider variety of food preferences and allergies.) Ever since, I've incorporated fish and seafood into my diet albeit like many pescatarians, with certain restrictions based on taste, texture, health, and sustainability. (Note that from here on I will use the word "fish" to refer to both finned fish like tuna, sole, and salmon, as well as seafood such as crab, shrimp, lobster, and scallops.)

The pescatarian diet could be terrific for you if, like me, you prefer to avoid meat but want the option of eating fish, eggs, and dairy. Moreover, the beauty of this diet is that, regardless of whether you decide to become vegetarian or vegan next, removing meat from your plate is the single most effective action you can take to vastly improve your health, the well-being of the environment, and animal welfare.

Yet as with any plant-based diet, there are nuances to pescatarian eating that are important to understand as you craft your new dietary habits. For instance, whereas I only eat fresh (non-frozen), local fish, usually flaky white varieties such as sole or fluke and seafood such as shrimp, crab, lobster, scallops, and occasionally wild salmon, you might prefer saltier fish like sardines, meatier fish like tuna, or organic (aka farm-raised) Atlantic salmon. Convenience, cost, and where you live might additionally drive you to choose frozen over fresh.

There are also particular challenges to removing meat entirely from a diet. Meat has a unique texture, umami flavor, and satiation factor, none of which is easily replicated. Because the body can become reliant on these distinctive facets of meat, when you start getting rid of it, you might experience internal resistance in the form of cravings. The information in this section will assist you in making smart choices about what types of fish and vegetables you substitute for meat, as well as in tackling some common obstacles that arise when one gives up meat entirely.

After salt, sweet, bitter, and sour, umami is the fifth category of taste, commonly known as savory. In Japanese, it literally means "deliciousness." Umami stimulates distinct savory taste receptors, which respond to glutamates. Glutamates, also known as MSG, are frequently inherent in or added to protein-rich foods such as meat. Some fish such as cod, shrimp, scallops, sardines, and anchovies contain umami too, as do some vegetables such as mushrooms, ripe tomatoes, and Chinese cabbage. Of course, the ultimate flavor of any food results from a combination of factors specific to each food type.

How to Become Pescatarian: Steps and Implementation

1. **Adopt Meatless Mondays.** Even with the knowledge that fish is healthier than meat for humans and the planet, giving meat up entirely is still difficult for many. Why? Habits are hard to break. But being part of a movement can help secure your commitment to a new diet by reminding you of all the good things that come out of your efforts. Joining the Meatless Monday movement is an easy and structured way to dip your toes into meat-free eating, with the benefit of community support that has shown to facilitate changes in dietary routines. Meatless Monday, developed in

2003 by the Johns Hopkins Bloomberg School of Public Health and The Monday Campaigns, is an initiative that encourages the mass reduction of meat consumption for health and environmental reasons through a collective weekly commitment to one day of meat-free eating. And it has worked: meat consumption levels in the United States are currently the lowest they have been since the 1950s, which is in part due to advocacy efforts like Meatless Mondays. In 2012, Los Angeles became the first city in America to endorse citywide observance of Meatless Monday, which included adopting meatless meals in one hundred schools. Many other public-school districts from San Diego to Baltimore to New York (as of 2020, all 1,800 of New York City's public schools are on board), and universities such as Yale, Franklin & Marshall, University of Maryland, and University of California Santa Cruz have followed suit and participate in this weekly celebration, as do countless restaurants and bloggers. Meatless Mondays have gained so much momentum that they are now an international phenomenon: in Taiwan they are known as Green Monday and in South Africa as Meat-Free Monday.

Implementation: Every Monday, commit to eating completely vegetarian. Draw on the support of the online community for recipes and solidarity and bring the excitement of the movement home to your family, who will hopefully be up for trying something new one day a week. Experiment with going out and eating completely vegetarian, or try to find restaurants in your area that actually observe Meatless Mondays themselves and see what their menus are like. Spread the word to friends and colleagues to pique their interest.

2. **Decide which types of fish you want to include in your diet.** The sea world is incredibly diverse in what it has to offer our palates. From flavor to texture to color, big fish to small fish, crustaceans to mollusks, our oceans, rivers, and lakes are expansive playgrounds. That said, certain varieties of fish are healthier than others. Some fish like salmon are high in nutritious omega-3s, while others like swordfish are high in harmful substances like mercury. In addition, overfishing is an enormous problem of the aquaculture industry, so if you are concerned about sustainability of the marine environment, it's a good idea to stay away from species at risk of extinction.

Implementation: Get to know the fish you plan to eat and how often is considered safe to eat it. Below is a list of commonly consumed varieties, which can help guide you in how to include them in your meal planning. I have flagged the regional sources of certain fish to indicate areas that qualify as "best choice" for sustainability according to the Monterey Bay Aquarium Seafood Watch (a respected independent source of seafood information for consumers).

- Fish considered healthy to eat two to three times per week and that are high in omega-3s include:

Salmon (Pacific)	Lake trout
Sardines (Pacific)	Herring (high in
Flounder	saturated fat)
Sole	Canned light tuna
Hake	Anchovies
Haddock	Oysters
Shrimp (United States	Black sea bass
and Canada, but not	Scallops
imported)	Squid
Atlantic mackerel	Clam
Crab (Pacific)	Plaice
Cod (Pacific)	Pollock

- Fish that are overfished or endangered but are considered okay to eat one serving of per week include:

Atlantic halibut	Atlantic cod
Monkfish	Skate
Blue fin tuna	Eel
Chilean sea bass	Lobster
Atlantic salmon	Mahi mahi

- Fish that are high in mercury that you should consume very infrequently (a couple to a few times per year) include:

King mackerel (high in	Swordfish (imported)
saturated fat)	Tuna steak (bigeye
Marlin (imported)	imported longline)
Shark	Tilefish

MERCURY EXPLAINED

Mercury is a neurotoxin, which, in excessive amounts, can cause brain, kidney, and developmental problems in humans. Polychlorinated biphenyls (PCBs) and dioxins are toxic chemicals that usually enter the marine ecosystem as pollutants from thermal and industrial processing land runoff (and some natural events like volcanic eruptions and forest fires emit them as well). When fish (and other land animals) eat them, usually in contaminated feed, their fatty tissue absorbs the chemicals. Then, when humans consume them, they have the potential to cause adverse effects on our nervous, endocrine, and reproductive systems, not to mention cancer. While you should limit your intake of fish known to have higher levels of mercury, PCBS, and dioxins, these contaminants should not impel you to avoid all seafood, because they only appear in the food chain in trace amounts. More people die from heart disease due to a meat-heavy diet than any cause related to toxic chemicals that appear in seafood. That said, pregnant women and infants have a higher capacity to absorb these chemicals than the average person and therefore should be much more vigilant about avoiding them.

3. **Eat at least eight ounces of fish per week (based on a 2,000 calorie diet) in order to get the heart-healthy benefits of it.** Most Americans eat far less than the recommended amount of fish. According to the USDA, fish made up only 5 percent of protein consumed in 2014, compared to the suggested 20 percent. Moreover, studies indicate that one third of Americans eat seafood only once a week and half consume it occasionally—a couple of times a month or not at all. In order to get at least fifty milligrams of omega-3 fatty acids, which research shows improves heart health, *The USDA 2015–2020 Dietary Guidelines for Americans* recommends eating at least two 3.5-to-4-ounce servings of fish per week (one serving is about the size of the palm of your hand). Since you're no longer eating meat, however—and some experts agree that consumption of fish up to four times a week is also a reliably safe amount—you can feel comfortable eating more. (Traditional Okinawans, whose diets and longevity are lauded in *The Blue Zones*—see page 11—generally eat fish three times a week on average.) Expert analyses and reports by the Environmental Protection Agency, the Food and Drug Administration, and the Institute of Medicine conclude that evidence is lacking to suggest an upper limitation of fish intake for adults.

Implementation: Write down your goal of how much fish you would like to eat. Then look at your calendar and establish a weekly meal plan. Simply shade the days, meals, and serving sizes of fish you plan to eat, as well as which kinds using the above lists as guides. (For inspiration on how to prepare them, check out tip 6 and my fish recipes in this book.)

EAT FISH FOR A MORE HEALTHY HEART

A multitude of observational studies and randomized controlled trials found that participants who ate fish more than four times a week had a 22 percent lower risk of coronary heart disease overall versus those who ate fish less than once a month. If you decide to up your intake to more than twice a week, just make sure to consume a variety primarily from the first group.

4. **Learn about the aquaculture industry and its sustainability practices.** Sustainability in aquaculture refers to the longevity of fish stocks through prevention of overfishing, the impact of fishing on marine environments and essential habitats, the effectiveness with which fisheries manage their operations, and the social and economic impact of the industry on communities from which seafood is sourced. In addition, sustainability is often viewed through the lens of the words "organic" (otherwise known as farm-raised), "wild," "local," and "imported." Notably, some people consider farm-raised fish most desirable, while others strongly prefer wild fish and vice versa. The same goes for local and imported. There are upsides and downsides to each perspective.

   Implementation: Learn the definitions of the key words listed below so you can be informed about the fish that ends up on your plate. Once you are familiar with this vocabulary, download your state's Monterey Bay Seafood Watch Guide. This guide ranks the available fish where you live according to sustainability and will help you understand which are best and worst to eat in your location. If you want to delve deeper, you can also research eco-certifications. Other helpful guides on aquaculture sustainability you can consult include: Ocean Wise, the Environmental Defense Fund Food Selector, and the World Wildlife Fund Seafood Guides.

- *Organic/Farmed:* In aquaculture, "organic" refers to farm-raised fish. Rather than being free to roam natural bodies of water, these fish are confined to man-made tanks on land or in pens (made of wooden mesh, or net screens) submerged in oceans, lakes, and rivers. (The word organic is in quotes because, unlike with meat, there is yet to be a federal designation of it in the aquaculture industry.) Fish farmers, also known as aquaculturists, breed, raise, and harvest these fish for consumption by highly controlling their environments and what they consume. On farms, farmers generally serve fish the same feed—grains and soy—every day. Whereas some marine farmers maintain high-quality farms to ensure human health and restoration of endangered species, others engage in low-quality practices, prioritizing quantity, sales, and profit control over sustainability. Compared to wild fish, farmed varieties are cheaper, more widely available, and can contain higher amounts of omega-3s. However, the low-quality aquaculture practices in which some farmers engage are responsible for a host of negative consequences including overcrowding of pens; subpar feed made with animal waste, wild fish meal, and excess saturated fat; contamination by pesticides and PCBs; and the use of antibiotics and medication to prevent disease. So, if you are going to eat "organic" fish, make sure the farms from which you purchase it are run by conscientious aquaculturists who operate with high-quality practices.

- *Wild-Caught:* Like organic fish, consuming wild fish also has pros and cons for health and sustainability. Wild fish are free to swim and live in the planet's waters, eating a natural, varied, and nutritious diet, which appeals to many people. These fish are often less fatty than those that are farmed and contain far fewer synthetic hormones and antibiotics (some of these chemicals might enter their waters from human waste lines). But the lives of wild fish are not wholly glorious. Waste, fertilizer, pesticide, and insecticide runoff from land, as well as oil spillage, pollute their waters. When it comes to mercury, for example, which is spewed out of smokestacks during the burning of fossil fuels and then absorbed by the ocean, wild fish are often exposed to higher levels than farmed fish, whose aquaculturists make concerted efforts to maintain low levels of such toxins. Overfishing is another serious problem that comes with eating wild fish because it threatens the extinction of entire species. Not only do humans eat large amounts of fish faster than the fish can reproduce, but fishermen also use methods of catching fish that can disturb multiple marine habitats and life such as coral, as well as the marine biology ecosystem at large. Lastly, if you're going to eat wild fish, prepare to pay premium prices and search for them, as they are not widely available.

- *Local:* Usually wild (sometimes the terminology can include farmed), this term refers to fish caught by fisherman off nearby shores. The distance from the water to store is short, on average no more than forty miles. There are several benefits to eating local fish. By eating local fish, you can experience a greater variety of catch, which curtails overfishing of singular stocks. You will be purchasing fish that is fresh and in season, which in turn can help fisherman maintain business year-round. Through your seller, you can easily trace where, when, and how your fish was caught, which will enhance your trust in the product.

- *Imported:* These fish are either raised in one country and then transported usually by air or ship to another, or they are raised in one country, say the United States, then exported to another country to be processed, and then re-imported to the United States to sell. More than 90 percent of fish sold in this country is imported.

5. **Decide from where you're going to buy your fish and get to know your fishmonger.** Now that you have the knowledge to make informed decisions about what types of fish you are going to eat, you need to figure out where to get them. For many, grocery stores are the only option and are adequate so long as you know what to look for. Most big-box stores stock a range of frozen fish and many higher-end smaller ones also have fresh fish counters. Local seafood shops usually sell fresh catch from nearby waters—these would be your premium choice and your best bet for getting good information on the best fresh, seasonal, and local picks.

   Implementation: Look up what stores in your area sell seafood, then visit each one. Check out prices, label information, and certifications. If there is a fishmonger (and there often is one), introduce yourself to him/her and ask questions about from where their seafood is sourced, when it was caught, how it was transported, what the special catches of the day are, and what is in season. Purchasing in season ensures that the fish are harvested when they are spawning and plentiful (which helps preserve the overall population) and that you will be getting the highest quality fish of the moment. The larger supply of seasonal fish also means that your catch will cost less due to lower production and distribution costs. While in my opinion fresh fish is always best, don't be dissuaded from purchasing it frozen for price or convenience. Frozen fish can be a fine choice if frozen immediately out of the water and packaged well (look for vacuum-sealed, with a thick layer of ice, clear not cloudy eyes, and uniform flesh). The best frozen fish is, of course, also caught in season.

6. **Explore simple cooking techniques.** Many people are hesitant about eating fish simply because they are unfamiliar with how to prepare it. Little do these folks know that fish is one of the easiest and quickest foods to make, and there are endless ways you can prepare it, whether you want to enjoy a particular fish's distinct flavor and texture, or prefer for it to act like meat. Simple preparations that showcase flavors unique to each fish involve sautéing your fish in a pan, baking it in the oven, or cooking it on a grill with four basic ingredients you're likely to have on hand: olive oil, lemon, salt, and pepper. Hankering for a juicy burger? Choose salmon, cod, or ahi, which have a thicker, more meat-like mouthfeel and are conducive to forming patties. Fish is also a great, adaptable canvas for all sorts of ingredients. If you are in the mood for Asian flavors, you can whip up a quick soy-sauce-based marinade. If it is Indian night, break out your cumin, curry, and masala spices and add them to the cooking oil.

   Implementation: As you transition to a pescatarian diet, set a goal for yourself to learn the following six methods for cooking fish: pan-searing, frying, poaching, baking, broiling, and grilling. You can also try a couple of free online cooking lessons (from YouTube to blogs, they're everywhere), take a MasterClass, or follow a celebrity chef known for their healthy fare (e.g., Gordon Ramsay, Giada De Laurentiis, Jamie Oliver). If you're feeling a bit more ambitious, invest in a cookbook for more complex recipes or enroll in a class at a local cooking school.

7. **Use extra virgin olive oil.** Many pescatarians adopt habits from the Mediterranean diet, which is very similar. (The main difference is that the Mediterranean diet allows for small amounts of meat occasionally.) One such practice is the plentiful use of extra virgin olive oil when preparing fish-focused meals. Extra virgin olive oil is famous in both the nutrition and culinary worlds for a plethora of reasons. It is rich in monounsaturated fatty acids, which lower total and LDL (the bad) cholesterol, inflammation, blood pressure, and blood glucose levels. It contributes to HDL or "good" cholesterol, which is cardioprotective. It is also high in phenols, which are antioxidants that fight disease-causing free radicals. From a flavor perspective, cooking with extra virgin olive oil enhances the unique tastes of individual fish because of compositional changes that occur when the extra virgin olive oil and the natural fish oils combine (there is a bi-directional migration of the lipid components between the fish and the oil). The result is an enrichment of the fat in both the fish and the oil, which bolsters the overall flavor of the dish.

Implementation: Invest in high-quality extra virgin olive oil and perhaps more than one bottle so you can experiment with different flavor profiles—for example, have one variety with which to cook and one with which you can finish off your dishes; or try one infused with garlic and another infused with rosemary. A terrific resource from which you can learn more about olive oil is the official index of the world's best olive oil (www.bestoliveoils.com), which ranks the best olive oils annually.

WHAT IS THE DIFFERENCE BETWEEN REGULAR AND EXTRA VIRGIN OLIVE OIL?

Like other processed foods, regular olive oil is refined, meaning that it undergoes intense mechanical processing and heating, which, with the added use of chemical solvents, strips it of its many health-promoting nutrients. On the contrary, extra virgin olive oil is produced more naturally—pressed from ripe olives without heat or chemical solvents—which maintains its robust nutrient profile. If you are also wondering how and why extra virgin olive oil is different from other monounsaturated oils like soybean oil, the answer is that it contains phenols, which are particularly potent antioxidant and anti-inflammatory compounds that have positive effects on heart disease risk factors like cholesterol.

Is a Pescatarian Eating Pattern Right for You?

The pescatarian eating pattern could be perfect for you if you check the first two boxes below, plus any other box on the list:

- ☐ You've consulted with your doctor and dietician and are sure it is healthy for you.

- ☐ You want to give up eating ALL meat (land animals) but still want to eat fish, eggs, and dairy.

- ☐ You seek health benefits from eliminating meat from your diet. (See pages 6–7 for a list of health conditions that a plant-based diet can improve and information on the association between meat and disease prevention.)

- ☐ You want to increase your intake of fish and whole, unprocessed plant foods including fruits, vegetables, whole grains, nuts, seeds, and legumes, and would like to try experimenting with plant-based proteins like tofu, tempeh, seitan, pea protein-based meats (i.e., Beyond or Impossible), and natto.

- ☐ You are concerned about the environment and sustainability and want to contribute to preserving the planet through positive steps that reduce climate change.

- ☐ You are an animal-lover and want to reduce the suffering of at least some animals (and/or believe there is a difference between flesh of animals and flesh of fish).

- ☐ You enjoy eating out often.

- ☐ You have religious reasons that ask that you not eat land animals.

- ☐ You are potentially interested in stricter forms of plant-based eating such as vegetarianism and veganism in the future.

If you've checked first two boxes and any others, you're ready to become pescatarian. If you're still wavering on the second, perhaps you need to take some more time as a flexitarian.

Trivia

Q: Are fish and shellfish considered one of the eight most common foods to which people are allergic?

A: Yes, both fish and shellfish are considered among the eight major food allergens along with milk, eggs, tree nuts, peanuts, wheat, and soybeans. Unlike many other allergies that become known in babies and young children, fish allergies sometimes develop in adulthood. If you think you are allergic to a certain type of fish, you can find out by doing a skin-prick test, blood test, or an oral food challenge test with an allergist. (Allergy symptoms can range from mild hives and nausea to anaphylaxis.) If you are allergic to any type of fish, obviously, you should stop eating it—but you don't have to give up seafood entirely. It is common to be allergic to one type of fish but not another. Thus, if you discover that you have an allergy to shellfish or even to one kind of shellfish like lobster, it does not necessarily mean you cannot eat finned fish or other types of shellfish.

Q: Should pregnant women and children eat raw or undercooked fish or those that are high in mercury?

A: No. The Food and Drug Administration and United States Environment Protection Agency both advise against pregnant and nursing women, as well as babies and children, eating fish that is raw or high in mercury because foodborne microbes and toxins pose a particularly high risk to the fetus.

Q: Will I gain weight from plentiful use of olive oil?

A: If you are concerned about gaining weight from using too much extra virgin olive oil, I hope you can find comfort in knowing that despite their copious use of extra virgin olive oil, multiple studies show that pescatarian and Mediterranean diets commonly have a favorable effect on body weight. (People do not tend to gain weight by adhering to these diets.) That said, of course, you do not want to use extra virgin olive oil with complete abandon because each tablespoon comes with approximately 120 calories. So how much is safe to consume vis a vis weight? As long your overall diet is calorie and fat-appropriate for your body type, according to researchers who study the Mediterranean diet, up to four tablespoons per day could yield you the heart-healthy benefits of olive oil and will not put you at risk of packing on the pounds.

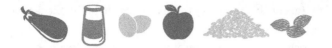

Diet 3: The Vegetarian

Vegetarianism is a diet rich in fruits, vegetables, whole grains, legumes, nuts, seeds, and plant-based proteins. It excludes all livestock and fish but can include dairy and eggs. On the surface, being vegetarian might seem simple; cut out all meat and fish and that's it, you're done—but not quite. You still have decisions to make with three common subgroups under the vegetarian umbrella. The first and most common subgroup is lacto-ovo vegetarian, which refers to those who keep both dairy and eggs in their diet. The second is lacto-vegetarian for those who consume dairy but not eggs. The third is ovo-vegetarian for those who eat eggs but not dairy. Often people subscribe to the lacto or ovo subtypes because they have an intolerance or allergy to either dairy or eggs, or think that one of these foods is simply unhealthy. But while some believe the more food groups you eliminate, the better off you are, research indicates that lacto-ovo vegetarians have the lowest coronary heart disease mortality among all the vegetarian subtypes. As someone who loves eggs and cheese, I've always made room for both in moderation, even when I was vegetarian.

Some people who are unfamiliar with this eating pattern worry that it can rob the body of essential nutrients. But studies show that well-rounded and well-planned vegetarian diets of all subtypes, more frequently than not, satisfy the body's macro- and micronutrient requirements, and can even provide a more robust nutrient profile than non-vegetarian diets. (Vegan diets are the exception, which we will cover in the next chapter.) Compared to omnivorous eating patterns, vegetarian diets tend to be higher in fiber, folic acid, vitamin E, vitamin C, magnesium, potassium, healthy unsaturated fats (monounsaturated fatty acids, or MUFAs, and polyunsaturated fatty acids, or PUFAs), omega-6 fatty acids, whole grain unrefined carbohydrates, and low-fat protein. Importantly, vegetarian diets are also replete with antioxidants and phytochemicals prevalent in vegetables and fruit. These compounds fight disease-causing free radicals in the body and attenuate the effects of harmful substances such as saturated fat (according to many studies, saturated fat intake is much lower in vegetarian diets than non-vegetarian diets).

As for concerns that vegetarian diets are lower in protein, zinc, and retinol, the average vegetarian intake of these nutrients is on par with that of non-vegetarians and deficiency of them is rare. The true nutritional risk for those new to this eating pattern is overeating the wrong foods, which ironically, can cause nutrient deficiencies. This is a problem for a subset of vegetarians who aren't in the habit of procuring, preparing, and consuming a variety of healthy whole foods, but who rely on nutrient-poor processed foods, which are excessive in fat, refined carbohydrates, sugar, and sodium. But don't worry—a focus of this guide is to educate you about the many healthful, satiating, fresh, and nutrient-rich vegetarian foods, and how to easily work them into your diet.

If health, disease prevention, and longevity are the motivation for changing your eating habits, you're in the right place. Research indicates that vegetarians tend to live longer than meat-eaters, because on average, they have lower blood pressure, total body cholesterol, and body mass indexes (BMIs), which yield fewer incidences of coronary heart disease, obesity, and type-2 diabetes. This in part has to do with the fact that vegetarians tend to eat a plethora of foods rich in soluble fiber like oats, legumes, chia seeds, citrus fruits, apples, barley, and psyllium, which also can yield a more balanced gut microbiome and a reduced risk of diverticular disease, IBS, appendicitis, and gallstones.

MACRONUTRIENTS VERSUS MICRONUTRIENTS

Macronutrients refer to proteins, fats, and carbohydrates. They make up the largest portion of nutrition we get from food and serve as the building blocks of our cells, muscles, tissues, organs, the energy that fuels our systems, and our brain. Most people who eat a balanced diet get plenty of macronutrients, and often even too many, which can lead to weight gain and obesity. Micronutrients are vitamins and minerals that the body also needs for optimal health and survival (e.g. metabolism and energy production, immune system, genetic transcription, antioxidants) but in much smaller quantities than macronutrients. It's more common for people to under-consume micronutrients than macronutrients, which can result in deficiency.

How to Become Vegetarian: Steps and Implementation*

Because most people who become vegetarian take the lacto-ovo route, the following tips are for this subtype. If you are a lacto- or an ovo-vegetarian, you can draw tips from this chapter and the vegan chapter.

1. **Embrace an entirely new category of food in lieu of meat and fish.** Until now I have hinted you should begin experimenting with vegetarian protein foods because they are both delicious and exceptionally healthy. (See pages 6–7 in Part One for health benefits.) Here, I urge you to deepen your relationship with tofu, seitan, tempeh, and legumes so you can make them a key part of your meal plan. However, rather than thinking of them as a "mock meat," I'd like you to consider them an entirely new class of food. By helping people change their mindset regarding these alternatives in this way, I have transformed many meat and fish lovers into vegetarians. By moving away from meat-centered thinking and plating, you too can start appreciating the unique textures, flavors, appearances, and smells of plant-based proteins, which will prevent you from feeling disappointed that you are not getting the "real" thing. The secret to enjoying this category of food is being able to appreciate its novelty, variety, and versatility.

   Implementation: With a little adventurous shopping and basic cooking skills, you can turn the purest plant protein foods into incredible meals. As you experiment with this new category you might encounter a disappointing meal here or there but if this happens, don't dwell on it or let catastrophic thinking make you determine that all vegetarian protein foods are terrible. Like with any new food, tastes change and are acquired over time so just scratch what you didn't like off your menu and move on to the next recipe. Patience is everything when transforming habits and lifestyle. Here are some ideas to get you started:

   - Canned legumes stored in water without added sodium are a great resource for quick, satisfying meals that don't require recipes or fancy equipment; try tossing chickpeas, lentils, cannellini beans, or black-eyed peas in a salad with leafy greens, tomatoes, cucumbers, and cheese, or in a soup, stew, or curry, or in a blender with walnuts, extra virgin olive oil, salt, and pepper to make a spread.

- For even heartier fare and when you have time, soak regular soybeans for a few hours and add them to soups and stews. Soy nut butter and soy nuts are also great for snacks and flavors enhancers too.

- Minimally processed tofu is a foundational food for vegetarians, and one they commonly cook and eat. Try my Tofu Satay or Tofu and Broccoli Curry on pages 252 and 246. Experiment with silken tofu, which can be a delicious base for spreads and dips, as well as desserts like puddings and mousses.

- Seitan, which is wheat gluten, is very high in protein, and has a texture that stands in well for poultry. If you love chicken piccata, try my Seitan Piccata with Kale and Quinoa on page 244. Or try an Italian flavored or smoky tasting seitan in the form of a kebab or ground in a veggie bowl, which in my experience, appeals to many transitioning to vegetarianism. Another of my favorite ways to eat seitan is in a simple taco for lunch with kale, a dollop of guacamole, and a spoon of chipotle vegan mayo.

- Tempeh is made from fermented soybeans that bind and are formed into a loaf-like product. More of the whole bean is preserved than with tofu, which gives it a stronger protein, fiber, and vitamin profile. Try my Eggless Caesar Salad with Tempeh Bits on page 187, Avocado Toast with Tempeh, Tomato, and Mustard Vegenaise on page 168, or Tempeh Stir Fry with Spinach, Ginger, Garlic, and Soy Sauce on page 238, which are super quick and easy to make.

2. **Get creative with eggs.** As covered in the flexitarian chapter, if you're free of diabetes and heart disease risk, you can safely eat up to seven whole eggs a week. Now is the time to squeeze the value out of this quota. With meat and fish off the table, eggs can move to the center of your plate at any meal, fulfilling your protein cravings and needs far beyond breakfast.

Implementation: Find recipes that make eggs the focus of your meal. Think frittatas (such as the one on pages 123 or 258), quiche, corn pudding, cheese soufflé, and other vegetable-based dishes like salads, toasts, cooked vegetables, noodle soups, and grain bowls, to which you can easily add a poached, hard-boiled, or over easy egg. Try my go-to salad with egg salad as the protein on page 181, soba noodles with a hard-boiled egg on page 236, or a veggie bowl topped with a fried egg.

3. Avoid excessive protein intake. Despite the range of protein choices available to vegetarians, including those described above, one of the most common questions for those transitioning to this eating pattern is still "Will I get enough protein?" The answer is yes, especially if you heed the guidance in the previous three steps to embrace a broad range of plant-based foods like eggs and dairy (both of which are complete proteins), legumes, nuts, tofu, seitan, and tempeh. In fact, a multitude of evidence shows that most Americans eat almost twice as much protein a day than needed, and even vegetarians consume about 70 percent more protein a day than the recommended daily allowance (RDA). Eating too much protein could result in excess energy intake (too many calories) and weight gain, which contribute to obesity and chronic disease. In addition, excess protein consumption along with not eating enough fruits and vegetables could result in weaker bones, because according to several studies, it could cause greater calcium losses in urine for a couple of reasons: 1) high-protein foods contain more acidic sulfur-containing amino acids, which are buffered by carbonates (acid-reducing bases) that can be leached from bone often along with calcium, which is also a buffer; 2) reduced calcium resorption (uptake) by the kidney, possibly because of an increase in glomerular filtration rate to eliminate the extra acidic amino acids and because calcium acts as a buffer to acids.

Implementation: Know what your protein Recommended Dietary Allowance (RDA) is and try not to exceed it by a large amount. The RDA for protein is .8 grams per kilogram of bodyweight, which on average for men is approximately fifty-six grams per day, and for women forty-six grams per day (based on a 2,000-calorie diet). It's easy to meet these requirements. A hard-boiled egg can have six grams of protein, a smoothie with one tablespoon of almond butter 3.5 grams, a cup of vegetarian chili twenty-five grams, a half a cup of Greek yogurt nine grams, and four ounces of tofu eight grams. In addition, eat plenty of fruits and vegetables, which are alkalinizing (not acidic), and especially those that are high in calcium, potassium, and vitamin C. Many studies also show that balanced diets replete with these nutrients can in fact be beneficial to bone health even with increased protein intake. (See Step 8 on page 89 for more on the relationship between potassium, vitamin C, and bone health.)

WHAT ARE COMPLETE PROTEINS AND WHERE DO YOU FIND THEM?

A complete protein is a food that contains all nine essential amino acids, which the human body cannot produce on its own. Amino acids are organic compounds that serve as the building blocks of protein. In total there are twenty amino acids that can bond together to form a protein. The human body can produce eleven of these but can only acquire the other nine through food. The nine are called "essential" because it is imperative that we consume them (our optimal health and survival depends on getting them). Some foods contain several amino acids and are thus known as "incomplete proteins," while others, mostly animal-derived foods, contain all and are known as "complete proteins." It used to be thought that if you were not eating a complete protein, it was necessary to combine certain foods in one meal to make one. Newer research, however, shows that if you are meeting your protein requirements throughout the day, you don't have to worry about eating complete proteins within a single meal.

Complete Proteins Examples: Meat, poultry, fish, eggs, dairy
Incomplete Proteins Examples: Legumes, nuts, seeds, whole grains, vegetables

4. **Minimize your consumption of highly processed and packaged foods, snacks, and desserts.** Overeating processed foods and consequently under-consuming vital nutrients is a main cause of malnutrition in the vegetarian population. Nutrient losses are substantial when food is processed (such as when wheat is transformed into white flour). Moreover, when transforming one food into another—for instance making seitan into a bacon-like product—food companies often add copious amounts of sodium, sugar, and fat to enhance flavor, texture, and appearance, which can have equally harmful health consequences. Processed foods include all packaged baked goods (think breakfast muffins and coffee cakes, Oreos, Twinkies, brownies, blondies, and gluten-free chocolate chip cookies and treats), refined pasta, white rice, white bread, boxed cereals, ice cream, and packaged vegetarian protein substitutes such as vegetarian sausage, wings, chorizo, Impossible and Beyond meats, and seitan-chicken.

   Implementation: Commit to eating whole and homemade foods as frequently as possible. If you can't make your meals at home, choose your market's highest quality prepared foods rather than those that are packaged and processed. In addition, refer to and apply tips 7 and 8 below. At the same time, give yourself some slack on a limited number of occasions when it makes sense to consume convenience foods. As long as you are eating whole foods most of the time, you need not worry about the few occasions when you're not. (I am a big fan of the "80/20 rule.") So, if you work full time and need to rely on a frozen Impossible lemongrass chicken skewer for dinner after a hectic day, don't beat yourself up. If you simply enjoy store-bought sweets on occasion, allow yourself to enjoy a muffin for breakfast once a week or a brownie or cookie for dessert every now and then (note that if you make these at home with nutrient-rich ingredients, you can enjoy them more frequently!).

ARE IMPOSSIBLE AND BEYOND PRODUCTS HEALTHY?

A critical aspect of adopting a plant-based lifestyle is reducing the processed foods you eat. Although these products are appropriate as transition and occasional foods on a plant-based diet, as with all processed food, it is best to abstain from making them staples of your diet. Composed of water, supplements like pea protein isolate and potato protein, soy protein concentrate, and flavor from heme in the case of the Impossible Burger, these products are a compilation of extracted and altered ingredients. In addition, both Impossible and Beyond burgers contain coconut and sunflower oils, which can be healthy in small amounts, but are high in saturated fat. Finally, as always, be mindful of what you eat with these dishes. French fries, Heinz ketchup, and American cheese counteract the benefit of healthier non-meat choices.

5. **Cease being carb-phobic (unless you have diabetes or celiac disease).** Low-carb diets have been around for decades—and they persist. But evidence of their success for long-term health and longevity for the general population is weak, and the notion that they yield sustainable weight loss is also dubious. The fact is that whole grains, which are carbs, are one of the most important staples of any healthy diet, as are carbs in vegetables and legumes. Why? Healthy carbs are the nutrient our bodies prefer to fuel energy output, because they are protein-sparing and break down into glycogen, which is the key substance that initiates muscular contractions. Furthermore, they are crucial to disease prevention because they promote a healthy gut microbiome and digestion, reduce

inflammation, and fight against numerous cancers. In a large study that looked at mortality, disease, and disability in 195 countries, low intake of whole grains and fruit along with high intake of sodium was responsible for the greatest number of diet-related deaths and disability-adjusted life years (DALYs). Specifically, low intake of whole grains was the leading cause of DALYs for men and mortality in women. Studies also show that whole grains assist with weight loss because they can increase metabolism and decrease absorption of calories during digestion. If you believe that carbs are your enemy, or that they are the main culprit of weight gain, it's time to reconfigure your perspective. Whole grain carbs are supremely healthy and should make up the greatest percentage of your caloric intake; 45 to 65 percent, according to the *2015–2020 USDA Guidelines for Americans*. (Note: If you have diabetes or celiac disease, this doesn't pertain to you and you'll need to follow a special diet. Consult with your physician and then a diabetes-certified nutritionist to work out a personalized diet that addresses your illness and suits your individual needs.)

WHOLE GRAIN LABEL READING

Ingredients on food labels are listed in descending order by the amount they appear. If the first ingredient listed is "whole," the product will probably be predominantly whole grain but if something else is first, then the product is not as high-quality, nutritionally speaking. It's best to look for a stamp on the package that says the product is 100 percent whole grain or whole wheat, which is reliable when the ingredient is listed first. You'll also want to avoid traps in the form of products with added sugar, salt, fat that are mixed with refined grains, and contain other unnatural ingredients. Try to avoid products that include words that indicate the presence of added sugars (such as "sucrose," "dextrose," "maltose," "barley malt," "rice syrup," and "high-fructose corn syrup"). Also use those labels to help you measure your sugar intake: you want to stay under fifty grams of added sugar a day. (Note that anything containing less than 5 percent added sugar is considered "low sugar" and more than 20 percent "high sugar.")

Implementation: Rather than eliminating carbs, replace refined grains with whole grains. If you do not already know the vast range of whole grains available, delving into vegetarianism presents a great opportunity to learn. There's quinoa, whole wheat, oats, millet, brown rice, bulgur, wild rice, buckwheat, kamut, spelt, and teff, to name a few. Instead of an English muffin, eat fresh whole wheat or whole grain toast, or my Three Seed Bread (see page 148). Replace Cinnamon Toast Crunch and Lucky Charms with my Homemade Granola (see page 133) or overnight oats (see page 139). Swap white rice with brown rice or any of the other above-mentioned whole grains. Try whole wheat, chickpea, corn, or spelt pasta, rather than white pasta, and almond flour tortillas rather than those made with refined flour. If you choose to buy packaged food, read all ingredients on the label closely to make sure you're getting what you want.

6. **Expand your vegetable and fruit palate.** According to the Centers for Disease Control and Prevention, in 2015 only 9 percent of adult Americans ate the recommended two to three cups of vegetables per day, and only 12 percent the suggested one-and-a-half to two cups of fruit. (One of the main reasons cited for this is the lack of access to fresh produce in many communities, the lack of time to prepare unprocessed, raw foods, and their expense.) In this step I am going to ask you to focus on eating not only more fruits and vegetables, but also a wide variety of them. This diversity is crucial for several reasons. Each fruit and vegetable type has a unique combination of vitamins and minerals that serve numerous functions from regulating our immune system (e.g. vitamin C, vitamin E, vitamin D, vitamin A, folic acid, selenium, and zinc), to ensuring proper cell functioning and growth (e.g. iron, potassium, sodium, copper, zinc), to protecting against disease-causing free radicals with unique antioxidants. Furthermore, some fruits and vegetables are associated with greater bone mineral density because they are rich in potassium and vitamin C. Potassium has bicarbonate precursors that have been associated with an alkalizing and strength-promoting effect on bone. Vitamin C is an antioxidant as well as a cofactor for collagen formation, both of which are crucial for healthy, strong bones. A cornucopia of brightly colored vegetables and fruits will keep your meals interesting, and your belly sated.

ANTIOXIDANTS IN FRUITS AND VEGETABLES

Carotenoids are important for normal growth, development, immune function, and eye health. Examples of carotenoids include:

- Beta-carotene: a precursor to vitamin A, found in carrots, mangos, apricots, pumpkin, spinach, and parsley.
- Lutein and zeaxanthin: abundant in green leafy vegetables like spinach, kale, Swiss chard, and mustard greens, as well as yellow vegetables like corn and yellow squash.
- Lycopene: found in tomatoes, watermelon, pink grapefruit, papaya, guava, and other fruits.

Flavonoids are particularly known for modulating the degradation of lipids, a process that results in cell damage and is involved in coronary heart disease and cancer. They are also inhibitors of LDL oxidation and have strong anti-inflammatory actions due to the fact that they are some of the most common antioxidant free radical scavengers. Examples of flavonoids include:

- Flavanones: found in oranges, grapefruits, lemons, limes, and bergamots.
- Anthocyanins: found in blackberries, blueberries, black currants, grapes, strawberries, eggplant, red cabbage, purple potatoes, and cherries.
- Flavanols: present in kale, onions, broccoli, and peppers.

Betalains inhibit lipid peroxidation, heme decomposition, inflammation, and dyslipidemia-related diseases such as atherosclerosis, hypertension, and cancer among others. They are prevalent in:

- Beets, rhubarb, Swiss chard, prickly pears, and some tubers.

Implementation: "Eating the rainbow"—taking in a variety of different colored fruits and vegetables—is the best way to ensure you are getting all vitamins, minerals, and antioxidants you need. Take time at the grocery store to browse the shelves and learn what is available and in season. Even better, visit a farmers' market or an ethnic grocery store where you will likely find an even wider selection of locally grown seasonal produce. Bring a notepad with you and write a list of fruits and vegetables you see and with which you are unfamiliar, or you rarely use. (Yucca? Dragon fruit? Fiddleheads? Kohlrabi? Rutabaga? Japanese sweet potatoes? Lauki? Palak? Parsnips? Turnips? Kumquat? Jackfruit? Persimmon?) This will help you remember their names and be a reference so you can look them up, learn about their special nutritional properties, and find cooking inspiration. Next, commit to buying at least one new fruit and vegetable each time you go to the market for a while. Then, when you get home do some research on how to prepare them. Lastly, take the foods you are used to eating and alternate them with ones with which you are unfamiliar. One way to do this is to stick to eating fruits in season when they are at their peak and most delicious. If you are used to eating berries every morning in the summer, come fall, try substituting them with apples, pineapples, and pomegranates. If your go-to summer salad incorporates tomatoes, cucumbers, avocadoes, and corn, in fall and winter include beets, carrots, Brussels sprouts, parsnips, and Jerusalem artichokes.

7. **Prepare ingredients and dishes in advance.** Because vegetarianism can be labor-intensive on the prep front, plan to use some weekend time to prepare for the week and even months ahead. The good news is that most fruits and vegetables will keep in the refrigerator for three to four days and many can be frozen for between three and twelve months. (The amount of time it takes for fruits and vegetables to go bad in the refrigerator varies from between approximately three days for most berries, stone fruits, and string beans, to one week for lettuce, tomatoes, and cucumbers, to up to two weeks or more for broccoli, citrus fruits, apples, and carrots.) Legumes canned in water without added sodium are a great staple to have on hand, but if you prefer to prepare them from scratch, once cooked, they too refrigerate and freeze well. Here are a few tricks that take some time initially, but save it down the road.

Implementation:

- Wash, peel, and chop your produce and prepare it for refrigeration or freezing. (Although recipes sometimes call for specific chops and sizes, you can easily prep ones you know you will use often, such as go-to salad ingredients and the vegetables in dishes you are certain you will be making from your meal plan.)

- Refrigeration of most vegetables is best when they are kept in the proper drawers and open containers with a paper towel to absorb moisture (but you must change the paper towels as they get damp). Make sure your crisper drawers are set to the correct humidity levels:

the closed setting is for produce that calls for high humidity while the open setting is for that which requires low humidity. Fruits and vegetables sensitive to moisture loss and ethylene gas belong in the high humidity drawer. (Ethylene gas is a hydrocarbon gas or plant hormone that regulates a plant's growth and development and the speed at which these occur. It is naturally produced when vegetables and fruit ripen and is responsible for their over-ripening.) Those that should go in the low-humidity drawer are the opposite—neither sensitive to moisture loss nor to ethylene gas.

- If you are freezing your produce, fruits can go straight into air-tight containers, Ziploc bags, or freezer bags once peeled and cut. If you are freezing vegetables, however, you'll want to shock, drain, give them an ice bath, and dry them before freezing. Because they get mushy upon thawing, frozen fruits are best used in their frozen state for smoothies, or immediately cooked down into stews or jams. Frozen vegetables are best thawed by being placed immediately in boiling water, in the oven for roasting, or in a sauté pan with cooking oil. If you go the pan route, expect some extra water to collect and simply pour it out into the sink.

- For legumes, if you prefer to make them from scratch, plan enough time to soak them for several hours or overnight and to cook them for at least twenty to forty minutes (some can take one to two hours). Then make the whole dish. You can store finished legume dishes such as soups, curries, and chilis in the refrigerator for up to a week and in the freezer for several months.

REFRIGERATION OF FRUITS AND VEGETABLES

High humidity drawer: Leafy greens, broccoli, carrots, Brussels sprouts, peas, cauliflower, cucumbers, eggplant, green beans, herbs, peppers, strawberries, and watermelon

Low humidity drawer: Apples, avocados, cantaloupes, honeydew melon, mangoes, papaya, pears, peaches, plums, nectarines, and apricots

8. **Buy groceries online or try a meal delivery service.** Cooking isn't for everyone, and that's okay. While it is always best to put some effort and tender loving care into what fuels your body, there is a world of healthy ways to get around the heavy lifting. Here are a few guidelines that can alleviate your meal prep workload.

Implementation: Select the service that best suits your lifestyle. If you work long days and nights, have kids, are in school, or just can't fit in time for cooking for any reason, this is your chance to take a deep breath.

- Grocery and meal delivery services, many of which cater to vegetarians, abound. Research your local area to discover the best resources. Fresh Direct and Whole Foods are great options for deliveries that include both fresh and prepared food. More affordable services include Imperfect Foods and Misfits Market, which sell "ugly" yet delicious produce at large discounts.

- If you have some time to cook but not a lot, or if you want to start gathering new recipes, meal prep kit services like Blue Apron, Hello Fresh, Purple Carrot, Hungryroot, Sun Basket, and Home Chef take a lot of thinking and chopping out of the process and all offer vegetarian subscription plans. These services provide boxes that arrive at your doorstep with the ingredients (sometimes pre-measured) and recipes for a set number of meals, for a set number of servings, from single to family.

- If you are looking for a more convenient way to get local produce, many farms now offer pickup and delivery, which increases the odds that your produce is fresh, and eggs and dairy hormone and antibiotic-free.

- And if you just want your meals made for you in their entirety, that wish can be fulfilled by companies offering ready-to-eat healthy vegetarian meal plans like Daily Harvest, Sakara Life, Zen Foods, and Provenance Meals.

9. **Consume nearly two times more iron than carnivores and omni-vores.** Iron deficiency anemia is not on average higher in vegetarians than in non-vegetarians, but vegetarians' iron stores can still be low and even inadequate for a few reasons. First, iron derived from plants is less bioavailable than that of meat (iron from plants contains non-heme iron, which is less absorbable than heme iron from animals due to plants' naturally occurring absorption inhibitors such as phytates, oxalates, and polyphenols). Second, some vegetarians, especially pre-menopausal women who lose iron during menstruation, simply do not consume enough of this nutrient (studies show that vegetarian men usually have adequate levels). Third, whereas whole grain products are vegetarians' greatest source of iron and they tend to eat more of these than non-vegetarians, it is estimated that more than 50 percent of phytate intake comes from whole grains and if you recall, phytates can block the absorption of iron. Thus, for vegetarians to successfully meet their iron needs (eight milligrams per day for men; eighteen milligrams per day for women between nine-teen and fifty years old, and eight milligrams per day for women older than fifty-one), they must make sure they are overcoming any of these potential obstacles.

> *Implementation:* Try to incorporate the top vegetarian sources of iron in your diet, which are beans and lentils, tofu, baked potatoes, cashews, dark leafy green vegetables such as spinach, fortified breakfast cereals, and whole-grain and enriched breads. Cook, ferment, and germinate your plant foods to enhance the absorption of iron from them, especially your grains and legumes (these procedures reduce phytic acid content). Eat vitamin C (top sources include citrus fruits, fresh squeezed orange juice, kiwi fruit, green sweet raw pepper, strawberries, broccoli) with your iron-containing foods such as fortified cereal or grains, because it too augments iron absorption. Drink less coffee and tea, because they contain tannins, which can reduce iron absorption. (When you do drink these beverages, try to do so a couple of hours after a meal rather than before or during.) Finally, because calcium can reduce iron absorption, separate the meals you eat to get these nutrients.

IRON DEFICIENCY

Iron deficiency anemia is the final and most severe stage of iron deficiency. It is when red blood cells shrink and fail to synthesize hemoglobin, which prevents adequate oxygen from getting to cells, tissues, and organs. The symptoms of iron deficiency include decreased cognition, fatigue, compromised immunity, pregnancy complications, and increased risk of lead poisoning.

Is Vegetarianism Right for You?

The vegetarian eating pattern could be perfect for you if check the first two boxes below, plus any other box on the list:

☐ You've consulted with your doctor and dietician and are sure it is healthy for you.

☐ You seek health benefits from eliminating all meat and fish from your diet. (Reduction of weight, type 2 diabetes, hypertension, cardiovascular disease, some cancers, and other chronic diseases and metabolic disorders are some of the conditions that can be alleviated or reversed by removing meat from your diet—see health benefits on pages 6–7.)

☐ You want to eat more whole, unprocessed food including fruits, vegetables, whole grains, nuts, seeds, and legumes, and want to increase your consumption of plant-based proteins like tofu, tempeh, and seitan.

☐ You are concerned about the environment and sustainability and want to contribute to preserving the planet through positive steps that reduce climate change.

☐ You are an animal-lover and want to reduce the suffering of at least some animals and fish.

☐ You may still want to eat other animal products such as eggs and dairy.

☐ You have religious reasons that prohibit eating any meat or fish.

☐ You are potentially interested in becoming vegan.

If you've checked the first and second boxes and any others, you're in the right place and it's time to get started on developing your new vegetarian lifestyle!

Trivia

Q: Is one cup of milk equivalent to one cup of other types of dairy?

A: For those of you who are lacto-ovo and lacto-vegetarians and keep dairy in your diet to ensure you get enough calcium (or because you like it), it's important to know that different types of dairy contain different amounts of calcium. According to the USDA guidelines, the following are examples of various dairy products that are equivalent to one cup of milk: 1.5 ounces of natural cheese or 2 ounces of processed cheese; $\frac{1}{2}$ cup of evaporated milk; 1 cup of yogurt; and 1$\frac{1}{2}$ cups of ice cream. As for calcium content, amounts can vary drastically even within each food type category: one cup of soft ricotta could have about 500 milligrams of calcium, while the equivalent amount of cottage cheese could have approximately 100 to 185 milligrams; six ounces of plain yogurt could have 300 milligrams calcium, whereas Greek yogurt 200 milligrams; eight ounces of milk has about 300 milligrams, whereas ice cream only has about 85 milligrams.

Q: Are soybeans legumes?

A: Yes. Soybeans are a type of legume. They are a species native to East Asia (many botanists believe they were first domesticated in China as early as 7000 BCE) and were introduced to the United States in 1804. Though soybeans share many qualities with other legumes—they are high in fiber, protein, folate, iron, and low in saturated fat—they are distinct because they are a concentrated source of isoflavones (see page 12). The soybean is one of the richest and cheapest sources of protein in the world and is a staple of people and animals everywhere.

Q: Should zinc deficiency be a concern for vegetarians?

A: While there is evidence concluding that vegetarians consume less zinc than omnivores and as a consequence might require as much as 50 percent more of this mineral (the RDA for men is eleven milligrams and women eight milligrams), studies also show that the average lacto-ovo vegetarian in developed countries has adequate zinc absorption and retention levels on par with that of non-vegetarians for two reasons. First, the body appears to adjust to lower zinc intake by excreting less of the mineral (which means it absorbs and retains more). Second, although many think phytates, which vegetarians tend to eat more of than non-vegetarians (in legumes), reduce dietary zinc—because they are in fact zinc inhibitors—modern preparation and cooking methods of phytate-rich foods such as soaking, heating, fermenting, and leavening minimize deficiency. On the other hand, zinc can be low in vegetarian populations from undeveloped countries due to limited access to foods rich in this mineral, such as animal products and whole grains. In addition, modern diets of these populations are often higher in unfortified refined grains, which contain lower amounts of zinc than whole grains (they are stripped away in the milling process along with many other nutrients), and lower in fruits and vegetables, which enhance zinc absorption. So, to answer the question, most vegetarians in developed countries do not need to think of zinc as a nutrient that requires special attention, but those in undeveloped countries can be susceptible to zinc deficiency. Some vegetarian foods that include zinc are baked beans, zinc-fortified cereal, low-fat yogurt, cashews, chickpeas, Swiss cheese, and oatmeal.

Diet 4: The Vegan

Eating patterns that eschew all animal-derived foods have existed for thousands of years in Buddhist, Hindu, and Jain cultures, among others. It wasn't until 1944, however, after nearly half of the cows in Britain were infected with tuberculosis, that the term "vegan" was coined. In light of this environment in which animal-sourced food could be tainted with disease, Donald Watson, a British woodworker, determined that a unique name was necessary for a diet that excludes two groups of food vegetarians commonly rely on—eggs and dairy—in addition to all other animal-sourced foods including red and white meat, fish, and any derivatives of these animals such as oils, powders, and chemical compounds. Although veganism is technically a vegetarian diet in the sense that both omit the consumption of meat, it has gained general acceptance as its own distinct eating pattern that is growing in popularity.

Many people who become vegan do so chiefly for one of two reasons: politics or health. Those who become vegan for political reasons are often referred to as ethical vegans. They adopt the lifestyle first and foremost out of compassion for animals (many also refrain from wearing leather and purchasing other animal-derived products such as leather bags and shoes, and cow-hide rugs). As for those who become vegan to improve health, studies show numerous advantages of this eating pattern. Like other vegetarians, vegans have a lower risk of heart disease, obesity, type 2 diabetes, cancer, and autoimmune disease than omnivores. Moreover, compared to all other eating patterns, vegans demonstrate lower body mass indexes (some studies show that vegans can burn more calories after meals than non-vegans because their calories are more likely used as energy than stored as fat) and fewer incidences of hypertension and hyperlipidemia. Finally, recent studies show that veganism can be beneficial to our gut microbiomes for two reasons: 1) the absence of animal products appears to increase the abundance of "good" protective bacteria and decrease inflammatory pathogenic microbes and 2) vegans have the highest intake of vitamin C, magnesium, fiber, and carbohydrates compared to others, all of which aid the digestive process.

As with any eating pattern, there are potential downsides to veganism. Due to the greater limitations of the diet, vegans can have difficulty finding enough to eat, especially outside the home. (While vegan food at markets and restaurants is more prevalent than it once was, many still do not cater to this diet.) This means that vegans may spend much more time researching, shopping, and cooking, which can lead to compliance difficulties and frustration. Vegans also must be extremely knowledgeable about the nutrient weaknesses of this diet and detailed in their meal planning to ensure they are adequately nourished. Research indicates that out of all the diets, vegans have the lowest intake and greatest deficiency of vitamin B-12, vitamin D, and calcium.

I can't help but close this introduction by being frank: a vegan diet is incredibly restrictive. The good news is that if you're up for the task—even if you try it on a part-time basis, such as one week per month, or eating vegan at home—you can reap the trinity of benefits we have been covering throughout this book: you can drastically improve your health, make a significant contribution to preserving the environment, and prevent the suffering and sacrifice of all animals slaughtered for food.

How to Become Vegan: Steps and Implementation

1. **Replace eggs and dairy with equally nutritious alternatives.** Assuming you've mastered vegetarianism of some kind, your goal for this eating pattern is to gradually eliminate eggs and dairy from your diet, making sure to compensate for the nutrients you could become short on with other foods and supplements (more on these nutrients in the steps below). Because veganism is so restrictive, paying attention to replacement foods becomes critical to avoid nutrient deficiencies.

   Implementation: Discover and use ingredients that can stand in for eggs and dairy and that will assist you in optimizing the nutrients you are forfeiting. Although your new lifestyle will take some time to set in, these tips will help you feel confident about the plethora of nutrient-rich ingredients and cooking techniques that will truly wow you.

- Plant-based milk beverages and yogurts abound these days in grocery store aisles. Experiment with several plant-based milks to find the ones you like most and for what purposes they work best (soy, coconut, almond, cashew, and oat are all very popular). In addition to using them in coffee, cereal, and smoothies, you can also use them as cooking and baking ingredients. But, make sure to learn the tricks of the trade. Plant-based milks do not act like dairy and work better in some dishes than in others, so use recipes (such as the ones in this book) to help you learn how to best incorporate them before you start experimenting on your own. In addition, as a vegan, you will likely benefit from fortified plant-based liquid products to ensure you get nutrients you will no longer be consuming in milk. (Learn more about plant-based milk beverages and view a plant-based milk chart comparison under "Trivia" on pages 110–111.)

- When baking, a common vegan replacement for eggs is a mixture of water and flax seeds (such as in my Vegan Chocolate Chip Cookies on page 277, which I love even more than my non-vegan ones). Craving fluffy pancakes or muffins? Baking powder (sometimes combined with vinegar or another acidic complement like lemon juice) is another miraculous ingredient that gives the light effect eggs often provide. You can experiment with my favorite corn muffins on page 153, or my whole wheat pancakes on page 145, which, with plant-based maple butter, walnuts, chia seeds, and flax seeds also provide a nice dose of protein, carbohydrates, omega-3 fats, and fiber, among other micronutrients.

- For casseroles and other recipes that call for eggs to bind other ingredients, some vegans swear by the egg replacer Ener G, which is made from potato, tapioca starch, leavening agents, and other chemical compounds. Other use agar and arrowroot. Vegetables mixed with ingredients like panko crumbs, grains, tomato paste or sauce, and water can bind without any egg substitute, such as in my eggplant meatballs on page 193.

- Just Egg is a solid vegan brand that comes close to getting the texture and mouthfeel of eggs right if you want scrambled eggs, omelets, fried rice, or frittatas.

- Feeling like a decadent bowl of macaroni and cheese? Vegans often use nutritional yeast mixed with garlic power, cashews, and other ingredients as an alternative to cheese for this dish.

- Vegan cheese made from cashews and tofu can satisfy a creamy-savory craving. (Pureed with water, they are also amazing as a stand-in for cream.)

WHAT IS NUTRITIONAL YEAST?

Nutritional yeast is a popular ingredient in vegan cooking because it contains protein as well as many vitamins, minerals, and antioxidants. It also has a savory, nutty, cheese-like flavor, which can help make some vegan preparations more satisfying. This type of yeast is specifically grown as a food product. Nutritional yeast comes in two varieties, fortified and unfortified. It is generally best for vegans to use the fortified variety, because it will bolster vitamin B-12 intake in addition to other key nutrients.

2. **Clarify and hone your motives.** Research indicates that cutting out food groups for intellectual (ethical, moral, religious, or spiritual) and social (ecologic, economic, or political) reasons might not yield the same health benefits as motives relating to physical well-being. Vegans, who exclude animal-derived products for intellectual and social motives, tend to eliminate food groups without complete consideration of how doing so will affect their nutritional status, whereas those who become vegan primarily for health are more likely to acquire the knowledge necessary to ensure they are eating an adequate, balanced, and nutrient-rich diet.

   Implementation: Read up on diet and lifestyle adjustments you will need to make in order to direct your vegan plan toward prioritizing your physical health and well-being. Make appointments with your physician and a dietician and use information from your exams and labs to learn the full scope of foods you will need to adequately fuel yourself. As a vegan, meeting energy requirements (caloric intake) is the most important nutritional component on which to focus initially, because calories in this diet are frequently a key indicator of whether you are possibly consuming the correct amounts of all other nutrients.

3. **Eat both raw and cooked fruits and vegetables.** While some vegans opt for a completely raw diet, fresh and cooked fruits and vegetables have distinct nutritional benefits, which means that including both in your diet will maximize the nutritional value of your intake. Raw food increases satiety, supports digestion, and normalizes gut transit time. At the same time, some fruits and vegetables are more nutritious when baked, sautéed, steamed, or broiled because cooking can allow for the release and greater absorption of several nutrients such as phytochemicals, which are otherwise bound in cell walls. For example, beta-carotene in carrots and lycopene in tomatoes are absorbed to a much greater extent from cooked vegetables than from those that are raw. Lastly, cooking vegetables may also reduce discomforts such as excessive gas and bloating that often accompany uncooked versions of the foods.

   Implementation: Unless you have a health concern or unwavering preference for one type or the other, consume both raw and cooked vegetables and chew them thoroughly. (Masticating raw vegetables is crucial in order to procure the full benefits of their nutritional value.) Take a few minutes to remember the following vegetables, which are more nutritious when cooked: spinach, mushrooms, carrots, asparagus, tomatoes, red bell peppers, broccoli, cauliflower, and sprouts. Next, make a point of eating them this way, at least some of the time.

4. **Take Vitamin B-12 supplements and monitor your levels.** Red blood cells, nerve function, and DNA synthesis are all reliant on vitamin B-12 for healthy functioning. Humans primarily get Vitamin B-12 from animals because it does not exist in plant foods. Whereas most vegetarians get adequate vitamin B-12 from eggs and/or dairy, vegans have a hard time meeting the body's requirements (RDA: nearly two and a half micrograms per day). Numerous studies show that absent supplements, approximately 86 percent of vegans would be deficient in vitamin B-12. A deficiency of this vitamin can cause symptoms of weakness, fatigue, tingling in the fingers and toes, constipation, loss of appetite, and weight loss, and can lead to pernicious and megaloblastic anemias, which can have detrimental effects on the nervous system.

Implementation: Take a daily or weekly vegan vitamin B-12 supplement. Vegan vitamin B-12 supplements are made up of bacteria and come in capsules for both daily and weekly use (i.e., 250 micrograms and 2,500 micrograms are common amounts, respectively, for daily and weekly intake. Note that only about five micrograms are absorbed from a 250 microgram supplement in healthy people). In addition to this, eat foods fortified with this vitamin (though be aware that the bioavailability of vitamin B-12 from fortified foods is uncertain, so they cannot be relied upon solely) such as breakfast cereals, soymilk, and nutritional yeast. A cup of fortified soymilk, almond milk, orange juice, or Kellogg's All-Bran Wheat Flakes could have six micrograms of vitamin B-12 (the amount will vary from brand to brand). One cup of fortified tofu could have about three micrograms. Finally, if you have any persistent symptoms such as heart palpitations, shortness of breath, numbness or tingling sensations, muscle weakness, and difficulties walking that arise as you become vegan, make an appointment with your doctor to get your vitamin B-12 levels checked.

VITAMIN B-12 AND FOLATE DEFICIENCY

Megaloblastic anemia is when a vitamin B-12 or folate deficiency causes red blood cells to become very large with underdeveloped inner parts, a malformation which signals bone marrow to reduce its production of them. Thus, in addition to the red blood cells being misshapen and defective, the body does not produce the required number of them it needs. Pernicious anemia is a form of megaloblastic anemia caused by a lack of intrinsic factor secreted by the stomach, which is necessary for the body to absorb vitamin B-12 and produce red blood cells. Because the body needs vitamin B-12 to produce red blood cells, those with pernicious anemia produce fewer red blood cells and suffer from weakness and fatigue.

5. **Eat plenty of seed and nut oils and consider a vegan algae supplement.** As a vegan, the primary foods that typically satisfy humans' needs for omega-3 fatty acids—fish, seafood, fortified dairy, and eggs—are no longer a part of your meal plan, which is why other sources of these important short-chain fatty acids must be staples in your diets. The three main omega-3s are alpha-linolenic acid (ALA), docosahexaenoic acid (DHA), and eicosapentaenoic acid (EPA). These fatty acids are essential, meaning the body cannot produce them and so we must consume them in our diets. ALAs can be acquired from seed oils and supplements. DHAs and EPAs exist in fish, seafood, and vegan algae supplements, and the body can transform small amounts of ALA into EPA and then DHA.

Implementation: For ALA, regularly consume flax seeds, chia seeds, hemp seeds, walnuts, soybean oil, canola oil, coconut oil in small amounts, peanut oil, and edamame. ALA intake requirements are 1.6 grams per day for men and 1.1 grams per day for women. On any given day you could easily meet your ALA omega-3 requirements with a smoothie or bowl of oatmeal containing one teaspoon chia or hemp seeds for breakfast, a salad with half a tablespoon of ground flax seeds sprinkled on top, and some vegetables sautéed in half a tablespoon of canola oil as part of your dinner. For EPA and DHA (each), make sure to take a supplement of 250 to 500 milligrams per day. Pregnant and lactating women should try to get no less than 300 milligrams per day of DHAs to support fetal CNS and visual development.

OMEGA-3s AND THE BODY

Omega-3 fatty acids, especially DHAs, are important for cognitive, immune, and cardiac functioning, and may reduce the risk of many diseases including heart disease, cancer, Alzheimer's, age-related macular degeneration, and rheumatoid arthritis. Additionally, the body uses omega-3s for energy and tissue growth, specifically for the brain, which makes them critical for fetal development. Several studies show that mothers who consume adequate DHA have babies with improved health outcomes compared to those who do not.

6. **Spend time outdoors in the sunshine and consume vitamin-D fortified foods.** The best sources of vitamin D for humans are sunlight, animal products like oily fish, meat, dairy, eggs, and fortified milks and breakfast cereals. Because as a vegan you will not be eating animal products, you need to ensure you will otherwise satisfy your vitamin D requirements. A lack of vitamin D, which is critical for the absorption of calcium, is also associated with weak bones and an increased risk of heart disease, cancer, and type-2 diabetes. Newer research indicates that vitamin D is also critical for neurotransmitter and nerve functioning, as well as cognitive and hormonal health.

Implementation:

- Spend at least ten to thirty minutes in the midday sun at least three times a week.

- Eat vitamin D-fortified foods like plant milks, cereals, orange juice, and mushrooms (mushroom powder has the highest amount of vitamin D followed by mushrooms commercially exposed to UV light, morels, and creminis).

- Take vitamin D supplements. Your goal? 600 international units (IU) per day. If you wanted to try to get the RDA in natural foods alone, you could do so by eating one cup of fortified cereal (40 IU) with one cup soy or almond milk (one hundred to 120 IU) and berries for breakfast, a half cup of Portobello mushrooms (roughly 300 IU) in your lunch salad, and a fortified soy yogurt for a snack (80 IU). If you decide to take a supplement, most brands sell capsules with well upwards of 600 IU (2,500 IU is a common dose), in which case you need not worry about getting it from food.

VITAMIN D FROM UVB RAYS

The darker a person's skin, the more melanin it produces. Melanin acts like a filter for UVB rays, which means that lighter skinned people can absorb more UVB rays from the sun than can people with darker skin who live in the same place. Because UVB rays initiate the production of vitamin D in the body, a darker skinned person would have to spend more time in the sun to get the same benefits (between thirty minutes and three hours). People who live in northern atmospheres where sunlight can be limited are also a greater risk of vitamin D deficiency and should be conscientious about getting it from other sources.

7. **Make a list of foods and their amounts that provide the same amount of calcium as one cup of milk.** As a vegan, milk is clearly no longer a source for fulfilling your calcium RDAs. (Men: 1,000 milligrams per day; women: 1,200 milligrams per day.) Luckily, dark leafy greens and beans are great alternative sources of calcium and we absorb twice as much of it from them—about 60 percent—as we do from dairy foods. Equally important to getting enough calcium in your diet is what nutrients you consume along with it, which is critical. Certain compounds such as oxalic acid (present in spinach, beet greens, rhubarb, and Swiss chard) and phytic acid (present in wheat bran, legumes, soy, nuts, and soy isolates) can decrease one's ability to absorb calcium. For instance, the difference in calcium absorption between foods high in oxalic acid compared to those low in this compound can be at least 45 percent (we absorb about 5 percent from high oxalic foods compared to more than 50 percent from low ones). Finally, protein and vitamin D increase calcium absorption, so meeting the recommendations for these nutrients will bolster your calcium levels.

   Implementation: Eat plant-based foods that are calcium-rich and well-absorbed by the body such as broccoli, kale, bok choy, collard greens, tofu set with calcium salts, and fortified foods like plant milks, orange juice, and cereals. Also make a list of the calcium-rich foods you plan to eat on a regular basis, noting which of them provide the same amount of calcium (or more) as one cup of milk (ninety-six milligrams of absorbable calcium). Examples of foods that contain equivalent calcium to one cup of milk include two tablespoons of almond butter or tahini, one-quarter cup calcium-fortified tofu, one-half cup fortified plant milk, two navel oranges, ten figs, and two cups of cooked broccoli.

8. **Develop your cooking skills at home.** Vegan fare can be complicated and time consuming to make. Unlike meat and fish, which can be delicious with olive oil, lemon, salt, and pepper, bringing out the flavors in vegan dishes often requires skilled use of herbs, spices, and sauces. Baking with vegan ingredients can be even trickier, because vegan replacements for common baking ingredients like milk, cream, butter, and eggs behave differently than their counterparts. (See page 100.) That said, there are many vegan recipes that are surprisingly simple and quick to make.

   Implementation: Enroll in a few vegan cooking classes in person or online. If possible, grab a friend or family member to join you because as with any new diet, support is a key aspect of success (and it can be more fun!). Browse some of the many vegan cooking websites such as *The Full Helping, MyNewRoots, Oh She Glows, Vietvegan, The Korean Vegan, Veggiekins, Jessica in the Kitchen,* and *Vegan Richa.* Print your favorite recipes and place them in a binder. This can be the beginning of your personal go-to vegan cookbook that will satisfy your need for variety and tasty food, and that will be amenable to your busy schedule. Organize your binder by meals, but use tabs to indicate recipes that are quick and easy so you can always find those.

9. **Restock your pantry.** Vegan food requires many ingredients most newly vegan people don't typically keep in their kitchens. Having a limited range of ingredients can make vegan meals taste mundane, but incorporating spices and seasonings will keep them interesting and flavorful.

   Implementation: Now that you have your binder, read the recipes again and make a list of ingredients you don't typically have on hand. Spices and herbs, vegan mayonnaise, nutritional yeast, plentiful legumes, seeds, and plant-based butter, oil, and milk options are some likely staples you will need. If you prefer to shop in person, do some research to figure out which stores carry these goods. Whole Foods, Trader Joe's, and smaller health food stores can certainly get you started, however, you may need to order some ingredients online. Amazon and FreshDirect have a solid selection of vegan goods as do smaller vegan grocers such as Vegan Essentials and Billion Vegans.

10. **Establish a list of restaurants at which you can comfortably dine.**
As a vegan, eating out can be challenging because many restaurant vege-table dishes contain butter and other forms of dairy and eggs. It will therefore help to have a list of restaurants near your home and work that are vegan or vegan friendly. Keep in mind that sometimes as a vegan, your best (or only) option when eating out will be to make a meal out of salads and side dishes. (Though do not hesitate to ask your server if there is anything off menu that could comply with your diet.)

> *Implementation:* Find vegan restaurants you like but also consider the palates of those with whom you will be dining out. Since your dining companions will not always want to be limited to strictly vegan restau-rants, scout places that can accommodate both types of diners as well. (Mediterranean, Middle Eastern, Indian, and Japanese restaurants often have vegan main course options, so seek those out if possible.) Once you've completed your research, enter your list of preferred spots in your phone so it is readily available on demand.

11. **Don't let cost be a reason to shy away from this eating pattern.**
Even though many people believe a vegan diet is more expensive than the others, this is debatable. Your costs will depend on how and where you shop as well as what you buy. Pound for pound, many vegan staples such beans, rice, cereals, pasta, potatoes, and bread can be much cheaper than a pound of meat. Beans for instance, are approximately one dollar per pound, whereas meat can cost three to four dollars per pound. If you plan well and do some analysis, becoming vegan could in fact be on your side as far as cost is concerned.

> *Implementation:* As with any diet, purchasing completely organic can raise costs. Although buying organic is great if you can afford it, it is not necessary if you cannot. For example, you can create a healthy vegan diet that is part organic, where you choose organic for the "Dirty Dozen" (fruits and vegetables that tend to be submitted to high pesti-cide use) but not for other produce. You can shop at a grocery store instead of premium stores like Whole Foods. Many grocery stores now have organic produce sections too and they are cheaper to boot!

Is the Vegan Eating Pattern Right for You?

The vegan eating pattern could be perfect for you if check the first two boxes below, plus any other box on the list:

☐ You've consulted with your doctor and dietician and are sure it is healthy for you.

☐ You seek health benefits from eliminating all animal products including meat, fish, dairy, and eggs from your diet (e.g., reduction of weight, type 2 diabetes, hypertension, cardiovascular disease, some cancers, and other chronic diseases and metabolic disorders—Review "Health Benefits" section in Part One on pages 6–7 if you'd like).

☐ You want to eat more whole unprocessed food including fruits, vegetables, whole grains, nuts, seeds, and legumes, and want to try experimenting with plant-based proteins like tofu, tempeh, and seitan.

☐ You are open to eating new foods and taking at least a vitamin B-12 supplement.

☐ You are concerned about the environment and sustainability and want to contribute to preserving the planet through positive steps that reduce climate change.

☐ You are an animal-lover and want to reduce the suffering of all animals.

☐ You have religious reasons that prohibit eating any animal products.

☐ If you've checked the first two boxes and any others, you're in the right place and it's time to get started on developing your new vegan lifestyle!

Trivia

Q: Are pregnant and lactating women more likely to be depleted in omega-3s than non-pregnant women?

A: Yes. Fetuses utilize a significant amount of omega-3s—specifically DHAs—for their central nervous system development (brain, visual, and cognitive development). Omega-3s are also needed to produce breast milk, which puts pregnant women at a greater risk of deficiency.

Q: Is a vegan diet too restrictive for high-performance athletes?

A: It could be but doesn't have to be. Vegan diets tend to be lower in calories, protein, fat, vitamin B-12, calcium, and iodine than omnivorous diets, but at the same time higher in carbohydrates, fiber, micronutrients, phytochemicals, and antioxidants. The most important nutritive component vegan athletes should attend to in order to meet their daily nutrition requirements and performance goals is energy balance (the number of calories one consumes versus that which one expends through physical exertion) because this is often the best indicator of whether a person is meeting overall nutrient needs. Due to increased energy expenditure, the effects of high performance (i.e., decreased appetite, increased musculature), and performance needs (i.e., greater endurance, increased muscle protein synthesis, weight goals), vegan athletes usually need to both boost their caloric intake and carefully select foods to meet other nutrient requirements. These days many top level and professional athletes swear by their vegan diet.

Q: Are plant-based milk alternatives equivalent to milk? Which plant-based beverages are best?

A: No. Plant-based dairy substitutes are fundamentally different from regular dairy products so do not be fooled into thinking they are nutritionally equivalent. As for which plant-based beverages are best, it depends on your needs. The following chart shows a comparison that can help you determine which beverages could work best for you based on nutrition information, but consider for what you will be using them. (You will likely want different ones for cereals, baking, frozen desserts, and cooking.)

Plant-Based Milk Alternatives

Nutrition Info (1 cup)	Organic Whole Milk (Horizon)	Organic Low-Fat Milk (1%) Horizon	Blue Diamond Unsweetened Original Almond Milk	Silk Organic Unsweet Soymilk	Oatley Oat Drink (The Original)	Pacific Hemp Milk	So Delicious Coconut Milk (organic unsweetened)
Calories	160	110	30	80	120	60	45
Total Fat	8g	2.5g	2.5g	4g	5g	4.5g	4.5g
Saturated Fat	5g	1.5g	0g	0.5g	.5g	0g	4g
Total Carbohydrate	13g	13g	1g	3g	16g	0g	1g
Dietary Fiber	0g	0g	1g	2g	2g	0g	0g
Sugars	12g	12g	0g	1g	7g	0g	<1g
Added Sugars	0g	0g	0g	0g	7g	0g	0g
Sodium	135mg	125mg	170mg	75mg	100mg	110mg	25mg
Protein	8g	8g	1g	7g	3g	3g	0g
Vitamin D	4.5mcg	4.5mcg	5mcg	3mcg	3.6mcg	2mcg	2.5mcg
Calcium	310mg	310mg	450mg	300mg	350mg	257mg	130mg
Iron	0mg	0mg	0.7mcg	1mg	.35mg	2mg	0mg
B-12	1.2mcg	1.3mcg	0mcg	3mcg	1.2mcg	0mcg	0mcg

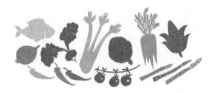

Part Four

RECIPES

Satisfying Plant-Based Recipes

The recipes that follow are designed to satisfy the requirements of each plant-based eating pattern and offer a variety of food, so that eating is always a fresh, fun, creative, delicious, and healthy experience. Some recipes were inspired by my own childhood favorites, others by my curiosity about different cuisines and ingredients, and still others by my experience as a mother, wanting to prepare healthy yet enjoyable meals for both my daughter and me. There is plenty to choose from: simple soups and salads for when you want something light or are pressed for time; plant-based versions of favorites like tacos, meatballs, and scrambled eggs; recipes for popular dishes like an açai bowl, chia seed pudding, and avocado toast. And you won't miss out on pancakes and waffles, muffins, or pasta—my recipes for all of these are included too, but instead of highly processed ingredients and unhealthy amounts of salt, sugar, and fat, the ones here are prepared with organic, nutritious ingredients, and tender loving care to ensure there is no loss of nutrition, taste, or satiety in any dish.

The next section also includes two sample weekly meal plans for each eating pattern, which you can follow as a blueprint for how to mix and match your own dishes and compose your own eating schedule. The meal plans are designed to be satisfying and to make transitioning between the different eating patterns easy for you. For example, the flexitarian plan includes only a few meals containing white meat to satisfy your omnivorous desires while also including some fish to prepare you for being pescatarian. The pescatarian plan includes more fish, eggs, and dairy to replace meat and prepare you for the vegetarian plan. The vegetarian plan relies more heavily on eggs and dairy for the nutrients you will no longer be getting from meat and fish and introduces more vegan dishes. Lastly, the vegan plan shifts the focus of each meal toward legumes, plant-based proteins, nuts, and seeds as substitutes for the animal foods from which you would otherwise be getting your protein, vitamin B-12, omega-3s, vitamin D, and calcium, among other critical nutrients.

Though some recipes are unique to each eating pattern, many meet the requirements of all. Each recipe is labeled to indicate which patterns they satisfy so if they fit your current goals, feel free to swap dishes as much as you like. The point is to have fun mixing and matching as you personalize your plan and make choices that fit your lifestyle.

If you get bored easily, you will likely want to have different dishes throughout the week at each meal. Since many people enjoy variety, I've primarily focused the meal plans on this approach. That said, an approach focused on diversity often takes more time to think about, plan, and prepare than one that is more routine. It can also make disciplining your intake more difficult.

If, like me, you do better with a habitual approach or are short on time and energy, I recommend you compose a meal plan with fewer options and more regularity. For instance, when it comes to breakfast, I usually have my Morning Antioxidant Smoothie most days of the week topped with my Homemade Granola, or along with a hard-boiled egg, Vegan Thumbprint Corn Muffin, slice of Three Seed Bread, or piece of Whole Wheat Zucchini Bread. Then on the weekends, I might treat myself to my waffles, crepes, oatmeal, or pancakes.

For lunch, I eat my Go-To Lunch Salad most days of the week (you will see this dish frequently in all the meal plans too), which I love because although the base ingredients are consistent, it has optional variety for certain ingredients. I usually pair my salad with a warm, plain almond flour tortilla on the side. When I feel like mixing it up, I swap with a soup and another salad, or other vegetarian dishes like my Roasted Sweet Potato with Sautéed Spinach and Cashew Cream.

Dinner is where I like to differentiate my meals day-to-day, yet for planning purposes, I often like to designate certain nights for a specific type of food. On Monday I might have fish, Tuesday vegetarian tacos, a pasta on Wednesday, and so on. The most important questions to ask yourself when you are designing your meal plans are: what is sustainable for your palate and health/nutrition goals, what is amenable to your schedule, and how will your plan affect your family or those with whom you frequently eat.

I have also included a few dessert recipes you can make with healthy unprocessed ingredients right at home. As mentioned in Part One, it's best to avoid commercially processed goods as much as possible. While my interests and chef skills are less honed for developing dessert recipes with whole, organic unprocessed ingredients, the internet and social media abound with them. Lastly, I also include some snack ideas for days when you need a little something to tide you over between lunch and dinner. These are entirely optional.

Acquiring knowledge and skills so that you can cook your food and plan your meals is half the battle of taking back control of your health and well-being. Applying what you learn to your everyday living with flexibility and balance is the other half. The most fulfilling win-win is when you complete the synthesis of all these things and your diet has longevity—when you no longer need to think much about your food intake, because your informed, personalized eating pattern and new refined habits will dictate your choices in favor of health and well-being. I wish you the best and hope you enjoy the journey of learning how to cook healthy and scrumptious food.

Key to Recipe Symbols

(F) **Flexitarian**

(P) **Pescatarian**

(VE) **Vegetarian**

(VG) **Vegan**

(VO) **Vegan Optional**

Breakfast Mains

Note: In the Sample Meal Plans (pp. 281–288), some of these recipes such as the smoothie and açai bowl are paired with those from the breads section to round out the meal, others with a side of fruit.

F

Turkey Bacon, Spinach, and Cheddar Omelet

My daughter is the quintessential flexitarian. She only eats bacon and white-meat chicken at her father's house or when traveling. One of her favorite ways to eat bacon is in an omelet along with spinach and cheddar. Though I don't usually keep meat in my refrigerator, maternal instinct drove me to perfect this omelet, so that if ever called upon, I could satisfy her bacon cravings for an indulgent breakfast on my watch.

Preparation Time: 10 minutes
Serves 1

Ingredients

1 teaspoon extra virgin olive oil
1 cup spinach
1 strip turkey bacon
1 teaspoon butter or vegan butter
2 eggs, beaten (plus one egg white, optional, for a more filling omelet)
¼ cup white cheddar, shredded
Salt and pepper to taste

Preparation

1. Add the olive oil to a medium sauté pan set over medium-high heat. When the oil is hot, after about thirty seconds, add the spinach. Sauté the spinach until wilted, about 1 minute, then transfer to a prep bowl.

2. Reduce the heat to medium, then add the bacon to the same pan in which the spinach was cooked. Cook the bacon until just before crispy, about 8 minutes. (Or if you prefer crispier bacon, an additional 3 to 4 minutes.) Transfer the bacon to a paper towel set on a cutting board. De-grease the bacon with the paper towel and then chop it into small pieces. Set aside.

3. Melt the butter over medium heat in a small nonstick pan. Add the eggs (and an extra egg white if desired) and reduce the heat to very low. As the eggs begin to thicken, using a soft spatula, gently drag the sides to the middle of the pan. Swirl the eggs so that they spread again across the entire bottom of the pan. Continue repeating these two steps until the eggs are mostly cooked through and set on the bottom, but not brown, and still appear glistening on the top, about 2 minutes.

4. Reduce the heat to its lowest setting (or turn off the burner but leave the pan on the stove). Sprinkle the spinach, bacon, and white cheddar evenly on top of the eggs. Place the lid on the pan to melt the cheese, about 2 minutes. Once the cheese is mostly melted, remove the lid from the pan. Using a spatula, fold the egg in half or roll it from one side to the other to form the omelet. Salt and pepper to taste and serve immediately.

Fried Eggs with Turkey Sausage and Avocado

While you've learned that it's best to nix regular sausage from your diet all together (see p. 22), you've also learned that white meat is healthier than red meat (see pp. 60–61). Therefore, if you're used to having sausage with your eggs to get you going in the morning, turkey sausage is a better choice than pork. Moreover, adding the avocado, which is rich in important nutrients such as folate, magnesium, fiber, potassium, riboflavin, monounsaturated fatty acids, and niacin, brings a crucial plant component to an otherwise all animal-product meal.

Preparation Time: 5 to 7 minutes

Serves 1

Ingredients

1 teaspoon extra virgin olive oil
1 organic turkey sausage, sliced into round coins
1 teaspoon butter or vegan butter
2 eggs
⅓ avocado, sliced into lengthwise ribbons
Fine grain sea salt and pepper to taste

Preparation

1. Add the olive oil to a small pan set over medium-high heat. Once the oil is hot, add the sausage coins and cook until browned, about 5 minutes, flipping the coins with tongs so both sides are evenly cooked. Reduce the heat to its lowest setting or turn the burner off, then place a lid on the pan to keep the sausage warm.

2. Heat an 8-inch pan over medium heat. Add the butter. When the butter is melted, crack the eggs into the pan being careful not to break the yolks. Cook to your liking, sunny side up (2 to 3 minutes), or sunny side down (flip the eggs). For runny yolks, cook the second side for another thirty seconds to 1 minute and then serve. If you like a hard yolk, cook the eggs for 7 to 10 minutes on a low heat setting so as not to overcook the egg whites.

3. Place the eggs and sausage side-by-side on a plate. Top the eggs with the avocado ribbons, add salt and pepper to taste, and serve immediately.

Egg White Frittata with Broccoli, Tomatoes, and Parmesan

Taking a part of something away from the whole can induce a psychological reaction of deprivation even if there are positive effects of doing so. I've seen this in people when they are presented with the idea of eliminating a yolk from an egg. Although yolks are healthy and contain the majority of an egg's critical vitamins and minerals such as vitamin B-12 and choline, there are times when eliminating them can be appropriate and beneficial: your doctor might have recommended you forgo yolks for health reasons, you might have reached your whole egg quota for the week yet are still craving a protein-rich meal, or perhaps you're allergic to yolks. (Yes, you can be allergic to the yolks but not the whites!) Regardless of the reason, if you are skeptical of a dish that appears to be missing a key component, I encourage you to try this recipe. Much of establishing a healthy eating pattern is about being adventurous and understanding that you can prepare food in myriad ways without compromising taste and satisfaction. Egg whites are extremely low in calories, at 13 calories per white, and because they're pure protein, very filling.

Preparation Time: 10 minutes
Serves 1

Ingredients

1 teaspoon extra virgin olive oil
½ cup broccoli florets, washed and chopped
2 tablespoons water
1 teaspoon butter or vegan butter (or olive oil)
1 cup egg whites (about 8 to 10 individual egg whites),
    beaten vigorously until fluffy
1 small tomato, washed and chopped
¼ cup Parmesan cheese, grated (or the grated cheese of your choice)
¼ teaspoon fine grain sea salt, plus more to taste
¼ teaspoon pepper, plus more to taste

(continued)

Preparation

1. Preheat the oven to 375°F.

2. Heat 1 teaspoon of olive oil in an 8-inch, nonstick, oven-proof pan set over medium-high heat. Add the broccoli and water. Place the lid on the pan for about 2 minutes. (This allows the broccoli to steam and maintain moisture), until the broccoli is bright green and most of the water has been absorbed. Then, remove the lid and continue to sauté the broccoli until its florets are browned and the water is completely absorbed, about another 3 to 4 minutes. Set aside in a prep bowl.

3. Reduce the heat to medium and to the same pan, add the butter (or olive oil, if using). When the butter is melted, add the egg whites. As the egg whites begin to solidify, pull the edges in toward the center of the pan with a soft spatula. Redistribute any liquid egg to the edges of the pan by gently tipping and swirling it. Repeat one more time.

4. Continue repeating these steps until the egg whites are mostly cooked through and set on the bottom, but not brown, and still appear glistening on the top, about 2 to 3 minutes.

5. Then, add the broccoli, tomatoes, cheese, salt, and pepper. Transfer the pan to the oven and bake until the egg whites are fluffy and completely cooked, about 6 to 8 minutes (Check by opening the oven and giving the pan a gentle shake. When cooked through, the egg whites will not move.). Add additional salt and pepper, if desired, and let cool for a few minutes. Slice the frittata as you would a pizza or cake and serve immediately, while warm. (Although it will sink a little once chilled, the frittata can also be covered and placed in the fridge for a day or two, then reheated or eaten at room temperature.)

Guilt-Free Spelt Buttermilk Waffles with Maple Butter

I am a waffle junkie, but the kind made with refined flour and topped with whipped cream, chocolate sauce, and other dessert-like ingredients that are often served at restaurants have never appealed to me. (And I don't endorse dessert for breakfast.) For a long time, I'd been afraid to test my hand at making baked goods and breakfast items with non-refined flour. But developing this recipe gave me confidence that many types of whole-grain flour bake beautifully, and can even produce superior results because their flavors are more complex than those of unrefined ingredients. The spelt flour in this recipe imbues the waffles with a very slight nutty flavor. (Spelt is an ancient whole grain, high in fiber.) Also, I noticed no difference when I migrated from refined table sugar to organic coconut sugar. Thanks to the buttermilk and baking powder, these waffles are as airy and nice and slim. Topped with a bit of homemade maple butter, you'll never be tempted by the diner again. If you make more waffles than you can eat, refrigerate the extra waffles for up to a few days. To reheat, preheat the oven to 325°F, then place the waffles on a pan and cook for eight 8 to 10 minutes or until sufficiently warmed through.

Preparation Time: 10 minutes

Makes 3 to 4 waffles

Ingredients

2 eggs
1 teaspoon vanilla extract
1 cup buttermilk
¼ cup butter or vegan butter, melted then cooled to room temperature,
    plus 1 tablespoon additional, chilled for topping
1 cup whole spelt flour
1½ teaspoons baking powder
½ teaspoon baking soda
½ teaspoon organic cane or coconut sugar
½ teaspoon fine grain sea salt
½ cup maple syrup
Special equipment: standard (not Belgian) waffle iron
Optional: berries for garnishing

(continued)

Preparation

1. Preheat your waffle iron.

2. Whisk the eggs, vanilla, buttermilk, and the butter in a medium mixing bowl. In another bowl, combine the spelt flour, baking powder, baking soda, coconut sugar, and salt.

3. Add the wet ingredients to the dry ingredients and stir until the batter is smooth. (Don't overmix; the batter should be combined but still look light and airy.) Let the batter sit for 5 minutes.

4. Grease the waffle iron with oil or butter of your choice. Pour about ½ cup plus 1 tablespoon of the batter into the center of the waffle iron (it will expand as it cooks to the edges). Close the iron and wait until the timer goes off. Open the iron and carefully lift the waffle from it. Transfer the waffle to a plate. Grease the iron again between batches.

5. While the waffle is cooking, add the remaining tablespoon of butter and the maple syrup to a microwave-safe bowl. Transfer the bowl to the microwave and heat until the butter melts, about 20 seconds. Pour the warm maple butter over the waffles, garnish with berries if desired, and serve immediately.

Scrambled Eggs with Avocado

Eggs are sneaky—they change shape on you quickly when you are cooking them. Scrambled eggs are no different: you have to constantly keep an eye on them, at every step of the process. First, the eggs need to be whisked so the whites and yolks are combined, but not overmixed. Once they are in the pan, you must stir continuously to the moment they are perfectly coagulated (solidified), but before they brown. This requires that you simultaneously keep an eye on the burner to adjust it as needed (you might need to turn it to low or off completely). Sometimes the most seemingly simple dishes require the most focus!

Preparation Time: 5 to 7 minutes

Serves 1

Ingredients

2 eggs
1 teaspoon butter or vegan butter
⅓ avocado, cut into lengthwise ribbons
Fine grain or flaky sea salt and pepper to taste

Preparation

1. Crack the eggs into a bowl and whisk vigorously until they are frothy and the whites and yolks are completely combined.

2. Heat an 8-inch nonstick pan over medium heat. Add the butter. Once the butter has melted, add the eggs. As soon as the eggs begin to set in the pan, start stirring them vigorously with a soft spatula. Keep stirring with vigor until the eggs begin to coagulate, taking a break for a couple of seconds every now and then so that they can continue to set. Continue stirring until the eggs are cooked to your liking, and not brown, about 2 minutes for runnier eggs, and 2½ for ones that are more well-done. Transfer the eggs to a plate and add salt and pepper to taste. Top with the avocado slices and serve immediately.

"Bullseye" (aka Egg-in-a-Hole)

This dish has been dear to me since childhood. When I was a kid, I loved the challenge of carving a hole in the bread, removing it without breaking the crust, then cracking the egg into it and frying it all up with plenty of butter. The results are irresistible—fried bread with an egg on it? How can you go wrong?—but the process of making this is equally as enjoyable (which is not always the case with cooking).

Preparation Time: 5 to 7 minutes

Serves 1

Ingredients

1 slice of your favorite toast, large enough to cut a hole 1½ inch wide
2 tablespoons butter or vegan butter, plus more if needed
1 egg
Fine grain sea salt and pepper to taste

Preparation

1. Place your bread on a cutting board. Take a glass or circular cookie cutter with about a 1½-inch circumference and press it firmly into the center of the bread until you hit the cutting board. Carefully remove the bread cutout so as not to break the surrounding bread and crust, and set aside. Heat an 8-inch nonstick pan over medium heat and add a tablespoon of butter. When the butter begins to bubble, add the slice of bread (without the cut out center). Fry the bread on one side for 1 to 2 minutes or until it becomes golden and slightly crisp. Using a spatula, lift the toast, add more butter to the pan if desired, then flip the toast.

2. Crack the egg into the bread hole. When the whites of the egg solidify, at about 3 minutes, flip the bread again, carefully, to avoid breaking the yolk. Reduce the heat to low and cook until the egg yolk is to your liking (2 to 3 minutes for a runnier yolk and up to 10 minutes for a harder yolk). When done, remove the Bullseye from the pan and plate it, yolk side up.

3. Using the same pan, increase the heat to medium-high. Spread the remaining tablespoon of butter on both sides of your bread center (the extracted hole) and place in the pan. Fry on both sides until golden, then place on top of your Bullseye. Add salt and pepper to taste, then serve immediately with a side of fruit.

Morning Antioxidant Smoothie

This is my go-to breakfast. When I'm pressed for time, have an early lunch, or am not that hungry in the morning, I'll have it on its own or with a couple tablespoons of my granola; if I need a heartier start to my day, I'll couple it with a slice of seed bread, a muffin, a slice of zucchini bread, or a hard-boiled egg. The strawberries and blueberries are full of antioxidants that power me through the day. The banana and almond butter provide many other nutrients including protein, fats, carbohydrates, vitamin C, vitamin B6, potassium, magnesium, and fiber, amongst others. You can use fruit that you've frozen from fresh at home, which is what I do, or you can purchase frozen fruit at the store. Evidence indicates that there's very little difference in nutritional value between fresh and frozen fruit and when and if there is, it's minimal. (After a year however, its nutrition will certainly begin to degrade.)

Preparation Time: 3 minutes

Serves 1

Ingredients

½ frozen banana
¾ cup frozen blueberries
3 frozen strawberries, stems removed, and cut in half prior to freezing
    (about ½ cup)
1 cup coconut water
3 tablespoons unsweetened almond milk
1 tablespoon almond butter (unsweetened, either smooth or chunky)
Optional: ¼ to ½ teaspoon organic maple syrup

Preparation

Place all the ingredients in a blender or Vitamix (Vitamix is preferred). Blend until completely smooth, with no visible blueberry bits. Pour into a glass and serve immediately.

French-Style Omelet with Caramelized Onions, Mushrooms, and Cheddar Cheese

Omelets are easy to execute but hard to perfect. How many times have you ordered one at a restaurant only to be served a rubbery browned version of what should be a delicate, tender, and sun-colored dish? Enter the French omelet, which necessitates a watchful cooking technique even more than its American counterpart because traditionally, it is filled with only cheese or fine herbs. This omelet preserves the French-style care in the cooking of the eggs, but adds flavor, dimension, and nutrients in its inclusion of caramelized onions and mushrooms. In both, the goal is to avoid overcooking the eggs and, as basic as this sounds, it's not so easy to execute. Eggs are impatient and will run to the finish line in the blink of an eye if you fail to pay attention to them.

Preparation Time: 10 minutes

Serves 1

Ingredients

1 teaspoon extra virgin olive oil, plus more to taste
¼ small yellow onion, chopped
½ cup white mushrooms, chopped
2 eggs
½ teaspoon butter or vegan butter
1-ounce white cheddar cheese, thinly sliced or grated
    (or another cheese of your choice)
Fine grain sea salt or pepper to taste

Preparation

1. Add ½ teaspoon of the olive oil to a sauté pan set over medium heat. After heating the oil for about thirty seconds, add the onions, stirring occasionally for about 5 to 7 minutes until golden. Transfer the onions to a prep bowl.

2. Using the same pan, add another ½ teaspoon of olive oil. Add the mushrooms and sauté until golden and crisp, about 5 minutes, stirring occasionally. Salt to taste and place in the prep bowl with the onions.

3. In a bowl, beat the eggs vigorously with a fork or whisk until they are frothy and the whites and yolks are completely combined.

4. Heat the butter over medium heat in a small nonstick pan. Add the eggs and reduce the heat to very low. As the eggs begin to firm, using a soft spatula, gently drag the sides to the middle of the pan. Swirl the eggs so that they spread again across the entire bottom of the pan. Continue repeating these two steps until all of the egg liquid is gone. Turn off the stove, remove from the burner, and place a lid on the pan. Let the eggs sit for about 1 minute, until the top is no longer runny, while making sure that the bottom does not brown. (You can carefully check the bottom without disturbing the eggs by removing the lid for a moment and gently lifting the edges of the egg with a soft spatula.) Then remove the lid and return the pan to its burner over very low heat.

5. Sprinkle the grated cheese over the egg. Place the lid on the pan again until the cheese melts, about 1 minute. Remove the lid from the pan and sprinkle the onions and mushrooms over the egg. Fold the egg in half with a spatula, or use the spatula to roll the egg and filling from one side of the pan to the other to form the omelet. Salt and pepper to taste, then serve immediately with a side of seasonal fruit.

Greek Yogurt Parfait

*These days supermarkets and high-end grocery store shelves abound with
Greek yogurt. While it takes some taste testing to find brand or type you like
most, when you do, a parfait is a nutritious breakfast option with which to
start your day. Among many other nutrients, it packs in calcium, Vitamin D,
omega-3 fatty acids, protein, fat, whole grain carbs, fiber, and antioxidants.
Moreover, Greek yogurt contains probiotics, which are live bacteria that are
extremely beneficial to our gut because they help balance the "good" and "bad"
bacteria residing in our intestines. When choosing a yogurt, keep in mind that
sugar content is as important as fat content: a yogurt with no fat but tons of
sugar can in fact be unhealthier than one with some fat and less sugar. Note:
this recipe can be made vegan by substituting the regular Greek yogurt for a
vegan alternative.*

Preparation Time: 3 minutes

Serves 1

Ingredients

4 to 6 ounces Greek yogurt, or a vegan yogurt
1 teaspoon organic maple syrup (optional)
½ cup Homemade Granola (see page 133)
½ cup mixed berries (blueberries, raspberries, strawberries, blackberries)

Preparation

Place half of the yogurt in a glass. Drizzle ½ teaspoon maple syrup over the
yogurt, if using. Layer half of the granola, followed by half of the berries on top
of the yogurt. Starting with the remaining yogurt, repeat all the layers again
and serve immediately.

Homemade Granola

This recipe harks back to my days as a yoga studio proprietor. Owning a yoga studio not only introduced me to an array of health-conscious students and employees, but also to the recipes that fueled their healthy lifestyles. One of my trainees who has celiac disease shared her gluten-free version of granola with me, which had been passed down to her from her mother. To this day, it's one of two granola recipes I make at home (though I usually go for regular rolled oats, not the gluten-free). I particularly love that it contains quinoa, almonds, and flax seeds, which bring omega-3s, protein, and other healthy nutrients to the table. The cinnamon and nutmeg infuse the granola with a lovely warming quality that screams of comfort food—but in a healthy way.

Preparation Time: 50 minutes

Makes about 5 cups

Ingredients

4 cups whole rolled oats, or gluten-free oats
½ cup uncooked quinoa
½ cup flax seeds
1½ cup almonds, chopped
⅓ cup coconut oil
⅓ cup organic maple syrup
1 tablespoon cinnamon
½ teaspoon nutmeg

Preparation

1. Preheat the oven to 300°F.
2. Combine the oats, quinoa, flax seeds, and almonds in a bowl.
3. In a saucepan over low heat, combine the coconut oil, maple syrup, cinnamon, and nutmeg. Heat until the coconut oil is melted and then remove from heat. Cool the wet ingredients to room temperature (slightly above room temperature is okay if you're in a rush).
4. Add the wet ingredients to the bowl of dry ingredients and mix well, until dry ingredients are evenly coated.

(continued)

5. Transfer the granola to a baking sheet and spread it into a layer, about ⅛ inch thick. Pat down the granola with a spatula so that it melds together (this will help it to form clusters). Transfer the sheet to the oven. Bake the granola for 20 minutes, then remove from oven, carefully rotate it with a spatula, press it down again, and bake for another 20 minutes, or until golden brown throughout. When the granola is done, let cool to room temperature before serving.

6. Serve on top of a smoothie, with milk or yogurt of your choice, or dry if you prefer.

Whole Wheat Crepes

This recipe is inspired by pfannkuchen, a traditional German crepe-like pancake I ate as a child. I've given them a healthy, whole grain twist by using whole wheat flour instead of all-purpose flour. I've also eliminated sugar from the batter because whole wheat flour brings its own sweet flavor, and I like to finish my crepes with sweet toppings anyway. Butter and sugar, maple butter, and strawberry jam are a few of my favorites.

Preparation Time: 10 minutes

Makes 3–4 crepes

Ingredients

½ cup whole wheat flour
½ cup almond milk, plus an additional 3 tablespoons
1 large egg
1 teaspoon vanilla
1 tablespoon butter or vegan butter
Optional toppings: maple syrup, maple butter (see recipe on page 125),
    cinnamon, butter, organic raw sugar, and jam

Preparation

1. Add the flour to a mixing bowl, then add the milk, egg, and vanilla. Whisk vigorously until the batter is smooth and very thin. (It should drip right off the whisk.) If the batter does not appear thin enough, gradually add up to a tablespoon more almond milk. (Sometimes it takes making the first pancake to know if you need more liquid.)

2. Heat a 10-inch nonstick pan over medium heat for about 2 minutes. When the pan is hot, add the butter and swirl it around to coat the pan as it melts.

3. Add about ¼ cup batter and swirl it around very quickly to cover the bottom of the pan until it forms a paper-thin crepe. (If ¼ cup batter is not enough to completely coat the bottom of your pan, add a tad bit more. If there's too much batter and the crepe is not thin enough, you can swirl the batter slightly up the sides.)

(continued)

4. Cook the crepe for about 1 to 1½-minutes on each side until golden and the edges start to shrink and curl toward the center of the pan (you can gently lift the edge of the crepe with a soft spatula to check).

5. Once the second side is done, transfer the crepe to a serving plate. Add your toppings to the crepe and then fold it in half twice so it looks like a fan.

6. Repeat the steps above with the remaining batter for additional crepes.

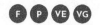

Vanilla Chia Seed Pudding with Cardamom

Despite their miniature size, chia seeds are essential nutrient powerhouses. One ounce of them (about 2 tablespoons) contains about 140 calories and is replete with protein (4 grams), healthy fat (9 grams), carbohydrates (12 grams), and fiber (11 grams), as well as vitamins and minerals. To make this pudding, you have to soak the seeds for at least a few hours or overnight (soaking the seeds results in a tapioca-like texture) but then it's just a matter of a couple of minutes to top them off and serve them up. Therefore, if you need to rush off in the morning, this pudding is a great, fast, and tasty breakfast option.

Preparation Time: Several hours to overnight, plus 3 minutes for finishing

Serves 1

Ingredients

1½ tablespoons chia seeds
½ cup almond milk
½ vanilla bean (or ½ teaspoon vanilla extract, but use vanilla bean if possible for optimal flavor)
Pinch cardamom or cinnamon (optional)
Optional toppings: 1 teaspoon organic maple syrup, ½ cup berries or other sliced fruit of your choice, a few crushed walnuts, toasted coconut shavings

Preparation

1. Add the chia seeds and almond milk to a small bowl or Mason jar. Split the vanilla bean down the middle and scrape the beans from the pod into the jar or bowl. Discard the pod. Add the cardamom or cinnamon if using. Stir the ingredients together until well blended. Cover the bowl with a lid or plastic wrap and transfer to the refrigerator. Let sit for at least 4 hours or overnight.

2. In the morning, stir the pudding to ensure it's well blended. If you're eating it immediately, drizzle the maple syrup over the pudding and top with the berries or other fruit, walnuts, and toasted coconut shavings. You can also store in an airtight container in the refrigerator for up to 3 days.

Poached Eggs with Pesto

Being creative with condiments will open up a whole new world of variety in your meals. The inspiration behind this recipe was my deciding, one morning, while poaching some eggs, that I wanted to add something to make my breakfast a little less plain. I pulled some leftover pesto out of the refrigerator and added it on top of my eggs. It was a great move: pesto and a runny yolk blend beautifully into a silky sauce (great for eating with toast), but if, like me, you prefer your yolks hard, it still provides an extra flavor punch as a garnish.

Preparation Time: 5 to 15 minutes

Serves 1

Ingredients

2 eggs
1 recipe Liguria-Inspired Pesto (see page 265)
Fine grain sea salt and pepper to taste
Special equipment: egg poacher

Preparation

1. Fill an egg poacher with about ½ inch of water. Cover with a lid and bring the water to a boil. Reduce the heat to medium. Remove the lid and crack the eggs into the poacher cups. Place the lid back on the poacher and let the eggs cook to your liking, 5 minutes for runny yolks, 10 minutes for hard yolks.

2. When the eggs are done, let them cool for a couple of minutes. Then using a spoon, carefully scoop the eggs out of the poacher cups so as not to break the yolks and transfer to a serving bowl. Garnish the eggs with about one teaspoon of pesto each, and add salt and pepper to taste. Serve immediately.

Overnight Oats, Swiss Müesli Style

This dish combines the preparation of the popular overnight oats with a century-old breakfast staple: Swiss müesli. Swiss doctor, Maximilian Bircher-Benner (thus the term "Birchermüesli," which it is also called by), invented müesli in 1900 at a health clinic. Once when I was in Switzerland, I couldn't help but ask a server what ingredients were in my delectable bowl of müesli. His answer provided the foundation for this recipe, which I've tweaked to suit modern overnight oats lovers, but also still includes the optimal ingredients and proportions that transport me to the snowy mountains or outdoor lakeside cafés of Switzerland whenever I make this.

Preparation Time: 2 hours or overnight
Serves 1 large portion or 2 smaller portions

Ingredients

⅓ cup plain or vegan Greek yogurt
1 teaspoon honey, or maple syrup if making vegan
½ cup whole rolled oats, gluten-free if desired
½ cup almond milk, or soymilk
¼ cup water
1 tablespoon walnuts, chopped
1 tablespoon golden raisins
Pinch of cinnamon
Optional toppings: ½ cup mixed berries, 1 teaspoon chia seeds,
    1 teaspoon flax seeds, coconut shavings

Preparation

1. Add the yogurt and honey or maple syrup to a bowl (or Mason jar) and thoroughly mix until completely blended. Add the oats, almond milk, water, walnuts, golden raisins, and cinnamon. Stir well to combine, cover with an airtight covering or lid, and refrigerate for at least a few hours or overnight.

2. If eating the entire portion, remove the müesli from the refrigerator, stir, and garnish with toppings of your choice. If you want to divide it into two portions, plate and garnish one, and keep the second portion in the refrigerator, covered for up to 3 days. (Wait to add toppings until just prior to serving.)

Morning Power Açai Bowl

According to lore, the now well-known and much-loved super fruit, açai, first came to the United States in the early 2000s. Southern California caught on to its nutritious and energizing qualities and it quickly became popular with local surfers. I was living in Los Angeles at the time and will never forgot the first time I tried an açai bowl in Santa Barbara, at a place near the yoga studio I frequented, steps from the ocean. I was instantly addicted. Açai bowls have since become prevalent from coast to coast, as well as on Instagram. I often make them for breakfast at home, because they pack in vitamins, minerals, and antioxidants, which give me a burst of fuel and delight as soon as my days begin.

Preparation Time: 5 minutes

Serves 1

Ingredients

2 blocks frozen Sambazon açai

½ frozen banana

¼ cup coconut water, or organic apple cider

Optional toppings: fresh strawberries sliced thinly, blueberries, fresh banana, frozen pineapple sliced into thin rounds, granola, coconut, chopped nuts, chia seeds, flax seeds, honey or maple syrup, cinnamon, walnuts, or nut butter

Preparation

1. Place the frozen açai and banana in a blender. Add the coconut water. Blend on a low setting stopping the blender intermittingly and scraping down the sides with a spatula as you go. (Given the small yield, this is not super easy in a large blender, so if you have smaller blender or smoothie maker, use that.) Once you have a relatively uniform purée, increase the speed of the blender until you have a completely smooth, but thick and spoonable texture.

2. Transfer to a serving bowl. Arrange your toppings over the açai and serve immediately.

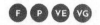

Steel-Cut Oatmeal with Cardamom, Cinnamon, Walnuts, and Maple Syrup

Like many people, I've been eating oatmeal since I was a kid. My siblings and I ate mostly whole rolled oats or quick-cooking oats, which were the kinds most available in the supermarket in those days. While these oat varieties are fine to consume on an occasional basis for recipes such as granola and müesli (which generally require whole rolled oats) or oatmeal on-the-go, the healthiest version of oats is the least processed steel-cut variety. Unlike their refined counterparts, which through processing have had the healthiest parts of the grain stripped away—the bran and the germ—steel-cut oats retain their bran and germ, which contain protein, fiber, healthy fats, B vitamins, phytochemicals, vitamin E, and other important vitamins and minerals. Although they take longer to cook, in my opinion, steel cut oats taste better in oatmeal than other types and have a nicer mouthfeel, plus I get great satisfaction out of knowing that I am fueling my body with unadulterated nutrient-rich food.

Preparation Time: 20 minutes

Serves 1

Ingredients

⅓ cup steel-cut oats
1 cup water
1 small pinch cinnamon (optional)
1 small pinch cardamom (optional)
2 teaspoons organic maple syrup
4 walnuts, broken into small pieces
Optional toppings: plant-based butter, chopped dried apricots, berries

Preparation

1. Combine the oats and water in a small pot and bring to a boil. Place the lid on the pot and reduce the heat to very low. Cook the oats until they are tender, about 18 minutes, stirring every now and then to ensure they are neither sticking to the bottom of the pan nor burning as the water gets absorbed. When the water is fully absorbed, fluff the oats with a spoon. Add the cinnamon and cardamom to the pot if using, and stir well to combine.

(continued)

2. Transfer the oats to a serving bowl and let cool for about 3 minutes. Top the oatmeal with the maple syrup and walnuts, add any additional toppings if desired, and serve immediately.

Tofu Scramble

Swapping scrambled eggs for tofu is a great way to serve up a protein-rich vegan twist on breakfast. Firm tofu mashed with a fork actually takes on a scrambled egg-like texture. Furthermore, the turmeric and saffron infuse this dish with a vibrant yellow hue and flavor reminiscent of scrambled eggs; if you didn't know in advance, you could easily confuse the two. Finally, this recipe is a basic palette onto which you can begin to fill your vegetable requirements for the day in all sorts of ways, by adding sautéed dark leafy greens like spinach or kale, or other scramble-friendly vegetables such as tomatoes, onions, mushrooms, or vegan cheese. Avocado and a warm almond flour tortilla on the side are two of my other favorite pairings, which, with a salad to boot, can also transform this into a satisfying midday meal.

Preparation Time: 5 minutes

Serves 1

Ingredients

Pinch saffron threads
1 tablespoon warm water
½ cup firm tofu
¼ teaspoon turmeric
Fine grain sea salt and pepper to taste
1 tablespoon extra virgin olive oil

Preparation

1. Add the saffron and warm water to a prep bowl. Mix and set aside for a few minutes.

2. Add the tofu to another bowl and using the prongs of a fork, mash it into a scramble, enough to get rid of any large chunks but not so much that is completely loses its form (it should look like fluffy scrambled egg whites). Add the turmeric and saffron-infused water and stir gently until the tofu begins to take on a golden hue (it won't show completely at this point, but you should see some color). Season with salt and pepper.

(continued)

3. Heat the olive oil over medium heat. Add the tofu and toss consistently for the duration of the cooking time, about 5 minutes, before it begins to brown or crisp. As the tofu cooks, you will notice the colors of the spices intensify. Salt and pepper to taste and serve immediately or let cool to room temperature, cover, and refrigerate for up to 2 days.

Fluffy Whole Wheat Vegan Pancakes with Maple Butter

For a long time, whenever I tried to make sweet breakfast dishes with whole wheat flour, I would end up with results that were unappealingly dense (the bran and the germ, which are stripped from all-purpose flour, remain in whole wheat flour, making it more nutritious but also heavier and denser because they get in the way of gluten formation, which typically gives baked goods their light and fluffy texture). As I learned about the properties of different ingredients and how they interact with each other chemically, however, I realized that baking powder can work wonders for the quality of whole wheat flour-based pancakes. Here, combined with the other ingredients, the baking powder does the magic of lightening the batter without the help of an egg, making the recipe completely vegan, refined flour-free, and sugar-free (save for if you choose to top it with sweet ingredients). If you are seeking to spruce up the nutritional value of your breakfast, choose your toppings accordingly. Flax and chia seeds, berries, and nuts can provide omega-3 fatty acids, fiber, antioxidants, and a host of essential vitamins and minerals.

Preparation Time: 10 minutes
Serves 2 to 4

Ingredients

1 cup whole wheat flour
1 tablespoon baking powder
½ teaspoon fine grain sea salt
1 cup unsweetened almond milk (or another plant-based milk, or buttermilk)
2 tablespoons vegan butter, divided
⅓ cup maple syrup
Optional toppings: additional maple syrup, berries, cinnamon, flax seeds, chia seeds, walnuts

(continued)

Preparation

1. Combine the whole wheat flour, baking powder, and salt in a mixing bowl. Add the almond milk to the dry ingredients. Whisk or stir well with a wooden spoon until the batter is smooth, but do not overmix. Let the batter sit for 5 to 10 minutes. This will allow the baking powder to react, which is what makes the batter light and fluffy.

2. Heat a skillet or griddle to medium-high heat. Add 1 tablespoon of the butter and let it melt. When the butter begins to brown, start adding the batter to the skillet, one spoon at a time (I like to make a taller stack of smaller pancakes but feel free to make the size you prefer). Cook the pancakes until the batter begins to bubble on top and the bottom sides are brown (carefully lift the edge of a pancake with a spatula to check). Then flip the pancakes and cook the other sides until those too are brown. Repeat this process with the rest of the batter.

3. Meanwhile combine the maple syrup and remaining tablespoon of vegan butter in a microwaveable bowl. Microwave for about 15 seconds, or until the butter has melted.

4. Plate the pancakes and top with the Maple Butter, or place in a bowl and serve on the side, as a dipping sauce. Add any other toppings of your choice, if desired, and serve immediately.

Breads

~~~

Three Seed Bread

If you've been keeping up with health-related news, I'm sure you've seen many articles on the gut microbiome and how important it is to optimal well-being. Our gut influences our brains, hormones, moods, and disease states—pretty much all of our major organs and systems. This means that we need to treat it well. Both soluble and insoluble fiber are key ingredients for a healthy gut. They reduce fat absorption and weight, lower cholesterol, decrease the risk of CVD, feed healthy gut bacteria, prevent constipation, and alleviate and reduce the symptoms and risk of many diseases such as diverticulosis, Crohn's, ulcerative colitis, and IBS. This bread is an easy, quick, and delicious way to get both types of fiber, thanks to the abundant seeds (flax, chia, sunflower), oats, nuts, and psyllium husk.

Preparation Time: 50 minutes
Makes 2 small 6 x 3-inch loaves or 1 large 8 x 4-inch loaf

Ingredients

1 cup raw sunflower seeds
½ cup flax seeds
½ cup raw almonds and/or hazelnuts
1½ cups rolled oats
2 tablespoons chia seeds
4 tablespoons psyllium seed husks (3 tablespoon if using psyllium
    husk powder)
½ teaspoon fine grain sea salt
1 tablespoon organic maple syrup
3 tablespoons melted coconut oil (place oil in a microwave-safe bowl
    and heat for 20 to 30 seconds, checking at the 20 second mark to
    see if the oil has liquified)
1½ cups water

Preparation

1. Add all the dry ingredients in a large mixing bowl and mix with a wooden spoon until thoroughly combined. In another small bowl, whisk the maple syrup, coconut oil, and water together. Add the wet ingredients to the dry ones and, using a wooden spoon, stir well until the mixture appears very moist and the dough is thick and adherent.

2. Transfer the dough to one large or two small bread pans. Using a spoon, press the dough firmly into the pans and then smooth out the top with the back of the spoon. Cover with plastic wrap and let the bread rest at room temperature for at least 2 hours.

3. Once the dough has rested, preheat oven to 350°F.

4. When the oven is hot, transfer the loaf pans to the oven on the middle rack. Bake for 20 minutes, then remove the bread from the oven and slide it out of the loaf pan onto a baking sheet upside down. (You can drag a small thin knife around the edges first to loosen the bread from the pan before you invert it.) Place the baking sheet with the bread back in the oven and bake for another 25 minutes if using small pans or 35 to 40 minutes if using a large pan. Let the bread cool slightly then serve immediately, while warm, for best results. You can also cool the bread completely and store it in the refrigerator for up to a week, or in the freezer for up to two months.

Whole Grain Almond Butter and Strawberry Jam Toast with Banana, Flax Seeds, Chia Seeds, and Walnuts

If you have followed any food accounts in the past two years on social media, you have likely seen myriad variations on creative nut butter and fruit-topped toast and here is mine. The most important step of this recipe is to hone your label-reading skills and buy the highest-quality ingredients you can find. If you recall, when buying whole grain toast, you want to make sure that the first ingredient on the list says "100% Whole Grain" or "100% Whole Wheat," or even better, contains the Whole Grain Council Stamp, which reads, "100% Whole Grain/20 grams or more per serving." If you see a package simply has the words "whole grain" printed on it, move on because such a product might only contain minimal amounts of whole grains. In the same vein, make sure to read the ingredients label of your almond butter. Look for jars that list "raw organic almonds" as the sole ingredient, and pass on the ones that include sugar, oils, and flavorings.

Preparation Time: 3 minutes

Serves 1

Ingredients

1 slice 100% whole grain or whole wheat bread
1 tablespoon organic almond butter (or another nut butter of your choice such as peanut, cashew, or sunflower)
1 teaspoon organic strawberry jam (or another jam of your choice)
6 to 8 slices of banana, cut thinly into discs
A pinch of chia seeds
A pinch of flax seeds
4 to 6 crushed walnuts

Preparation

Toast bread to your liking. Spread the nut butter over the warm toast, followed by the jam. Add the banana slices making single layer rows. Sprinkle your chia and flax seeds on top, then add the walnuts. Enjoy and serve immediately.

Whole Wheat Zucchini Bread

It's best to save store-bought sweet breads and muffins for an occasional treat because although tasty, they are usually packed with calories, fat, sugar, salt, and refined carbohydrates. This recipe, as well as others you can make at home with high-quality ingredients, is a healthier take on what you would get at the bakery or corner store because I've replaced white flour with whole wheat flour, butter with olive oil, and refined sugar with maple syrup. (You can also try substituting with coconut sugar.) Note: the optimal yield for this recipe is two mini-loaves. If you want to make a single loaf in an 8 x 4-inch pan, you will need to increase the cook time and watch and test the loaf carefully.

Preparation Time: 1 hour
Makes 2 6 x 3-inch loaves

Ingredients

Butter or vegan butter for greasing bread pans
2 large eggs
½ cup organic maple syrup
1 cup zucchini, grated on a box grater using the largest holes
⅓ cup buttermilk, or another plant-based milk
¼ cup extra virgin olive oil
1 tablespoon vanilla extract
1¾ cups whole wheat flour, plus additional for dusting pans
2 teaspoons baking powder
½ teaspoon baking soda
½ teaspoon salt
½ teaspoon ground cinnamon

Preparation

1. Preheat the oven to 325°F. Grease 2 small bread pans (or 1 large) thoroughly, making sure to cover all of the surface area so the bread doesn't stick to the pan. Lightly dust with whole wheat flour and set aside.

2. Crack the eggs into a large bowl. Using an electric mixer on a low setting or a wooden spoon, mix the eggs until combined and smooth. Add the maple syrup, zucchini, buttermilk, oil, and vanilla, and mix until those ingredients are combined.

(continued)

3. In a separate bowl, combine the whole wheat flour, baking powder, baking soda, salt, and cinnamon. Then, using a strainer or sifter, sift the dry ingredient over the wet ingredients. Using a wooden spoon, mix all ingredients until just blended (don't overmix).

4. Transfer the batter to the prepared bread pans and then to the oven. Bake until the bread is puffy, golden on top, and moist on the inside, about 45 minutes. (Check both at the 40-minute mark by sticking a toothpick or sharp knife into the center of the loaf; when ready, the utensil should come out moist but clean, without batter on it.) Take the bread out of the oven and let cool about 15 minutes before slicing. When ready to serve, run a sharp small knife around the edges of the bread to pull them away from the pans. Slice, and serve warm with jam, olive oil, or plant-based butter if desired.

Vegan Thumbprint Corn Muffins

I have a long list of happy corn bread memories. There were the mouth-wateringly delicious warm corn muffins that the deli down the street from where I grew up in Manhattan served up every morning, the honey infused Southern-style cornbread I indulged in over the decade I vacationed in Kiawah Island every Fourth of July, and then the mini raspberry corn muffins at Mary's Marvelous in East Hampton, which my daughter first fell in love with and then got me hooked on. As with all the baked goods recipes in this book, my primary interest in developing this recipe was to eliminate as many refined ingredients as possible, yet to also maintain the taste and texture of muffins that contain those ingredients. Although these muffins can last up to a week in the refrigerator and a couple of months in the freezer, they are best heated and served warm.

Preparation Time: 30 minutes

Serves 12 muffins

Ingredients

1 tablespoon flax seeds
¼ cup water
1½ cups spelt flour
1 cup fine corn flour (for a cakier texture) or cornmeal (for a rougher texture)
1½ teaspoons baking powder
½ teaspoon baking soda
½ teaspoon fine grain sea salt
1½ cups plant-based milk (i.e., oat or almond milk)
2 teaspoons lemon juice
⅔ cup maple syrup
⅓ cup canola oil
Optional: strawberry jam to fill the muffins

Preparation

1. Preheat the oven to 350°F.
2. Combine the flax seeds and water in a prep bowl and set aside.
3. In a large bowl, whisk together the spelt flour, corn flour or cornmeal, baking powder, baking soda, and salt.

(continued)

4. In a separate bowl, add and lightly stir the plant-based milk and lemon juice. Then add the flax seed and water mixture, maple syrup, and canola oil, and stir to combine.

5. Add the wet ingredients to the dry ingredients. Mix with a wooden spoon until well combined (some lumps are okay). Let the batter sit for 3 to 5 minutes.

6. Lightly grease the muffins tins, then add the batter about two thirds of the way up. If you're adding the jam, add a teaspoon in the center of each muffin (it will sink into the muffin when it bakes). Bake for 22 minutes, then test by inserting a toothpick in the center of a muffin. The toothpick should come out clean, without batter, but appear moist. Serve warm or cool to room temperature, refrigerate for up to a week, or freeze and reheat when ready to eat.

Pan-Fried Sourdough Toast

Sourdough bread is very popular, but, unlike many well-loved foods, it also has some nutritional advantages over other breads. If you have difficulties digesting regular and/or whole grain bread, sourdough is said to be easier on the gut. This is because its lactic acid bacteria from the fermentation process produce an enzyme called phytase, which pre-digests gas-producing phytic acid. If on the other hand the anti-nutrient effect of phytates is your concern due to increased consumption of legumes or other aspects of your diet (see page 14), these bacteria also lower the bread's PH, which helps degrade phytates. Whether freshly baked at home or purchased, if you haven't tried pan-frying your sourdough, this preparation is a must. The crispy yet soft glistening bread goes with virtually any soup or salad.

Preparation Time: 5 minutes

Serves 1

Ingredients

Extra virgin olive oil
1 slice sourdough bread, sliced about ¼-inch thick

Preparation

1. Pour the olive oil into a prep bowl. Brush the sourdough with the oil, coating each side liberally.

2. Heat a frying pan over medium heat. Transfer the bread to the pan and fry each side until golden and crispy on the outside but still soft on the inside, about 10 minutes total.

Lunch Mains

Note: Per the meal plans (pp. 281–288), these dishes are typically paired with soups, salads, breads, and vegetable sides to round out the meal.

Open-Faced Tuna Salad Toast

When I was young, my favorite lunch was tuna salad with Lays potato chips or on white Pepperidge Farm toast. This was back when packaged snack foods and white bread were in their heyday—and before trans-fat, salt, sugar, carbs, and processed foods were well-known enemies of a healthy lifestyle. Whereas it's perfectly acceptable to enjoy these treats occasionally, if you want to eat tuna salad more frequently, this recipe is the way to go. The oil-brushed sourdough toast is a healthier way to get a satisfying crunch, while vegan mayonnaise stands in as a lighter version of regular mayonnaise.

Preparation Time: 10 minutes

Serves 1

Ingredients

1 4-ounce can of solid white albacore tuna, packed in water
2½ tablespoons Vegenaise
1 teaspoon Dijon mustard
1 stalk (about 2 tablespoons) celery, finely chopped into very small cubes
Fine grain salt and pepper to taste
1 to 2 tablespoons extra virgin olive oil, for brushing on the bread
1 slice sourdough bread, about ¼ inch thick (or whole grain or sprouted bread)
1 leaf butter lettuce, washed
1 to 2 slices tomato, thinly sliced
1 tablespoon parsley, chopped (optional)

Preparation

1. Add the tuna, Vegenaise, and mustard to a bowl. Using a fork, mix to combine, mashing the tuna with the prongs of the fork until you get your desired texture. Add the celery and mix in evenly. Salt and pepper to taste. Set aside.

2. Add the olive oil to a prep bowl. Using a basting brush, liberally coat both sides of the bread. Transfer the bread to a skillet set over medium heat and cook on both sides until golden and slightly crisp, about 2 to 3 minutes per side. Remove toast from the skillet and set aside to cool to room temperature.

(continued)

3. Once the toast is at room temperature, spread the tuna salad on it. (Depending on how hungry you are, you might have extra tuna, which you can refrigerate and save for another day.) Then layer the butter lettuce and lastly the tomato slice(s) over. Salt and pepper the tomatoes to taste, garnish with parsley, and serve immediately.

Almond Flour Tortilla Flatbread

Almond flour tortillas are exemplary of how far the world has come in satis-fying dietary requirements of all kinds. They are gluten-free, vegan, delicious, and widely available in supermarkets and online. Having tasted several whole grain and white flour-free tortillas, I find their taste and texture to be the best of the lot. (For instance, I find chickpea flour tortillas and even some corn tortillas to be chewy and just not all that appealing to my palate.) Whether you want a simple quesadilla or creative flatbread like this, you will never feel cheated out of a white-flour tortilla. Although I use zucchini and Manchego here, you can use any vegetables or cheese you like (including vegan cheese). If you prefer to go cheeseless, the recipe works that way too.

Preparation Time: 10 minutes

Serves 1

Ingredients

2 teaspoons extra virgin olive oil, divided
1 cup zucchini, sliced into very thin coins (or any other vegetable
    of your choice)
Fine grain sea salt and pepper to taste
1 almond flour tortilla
¼ cup Manchego cheese, sliced or shredded (or another cheese
    of your choice, including vegan cheese)

Preparation

1. Heat 1 teaspoon of olive oil in a sauté pan over medium-high heat until it shimmers. Add the zucchini and sauté until golden, about 5 minutes on each side. Salt and pepper to taste and set aside in a prep bowl.

2. Using the same pan, reduce the heat to medium. Add the remaining teaspoon of olive oil and the tortilla. Cook the tortilla until you see golden dimples on both sides and it's crisp enough not to bend (be cautious not to overdo it, but you want it to be stiff enough to support the toppings). Then, reduce the heat to low, sprinkle the cheese evenly around the tortilla, and add the zucchini coins. Cover the pan until cheese melts, about 2 minutes. When the cheese is melted, plate and serve immediately.

Greek-Yogurt Chicken Salad in Lettuce Cups

High in protein, this recipe is guilt-free and a great way to satisfy your meat craving without overdoing it. (Remember 3 to 4 ounces of meat is an appropriate serving size.) If you like your chicken salad creamy, the Greek yogurt and dill dressing is a nutritious way to go. Rather than the saturated fat and cholesterol in mayonnaise, the yogurt brings in many essential healthy nutrients including calcium, vitamin B-12, phosphorous, riboflavin, protein, carbohydrates, and probiotics.

Preparation Time: 10 minutes

Serves 1

Ingredients

1 tablespoon extra virgin olive oil

3 to 4 ounces organic white chicken breast, diced into small pieces (or store-bought roasted white chicken breast)

1 celery stalk, washed and diced into small uniform pieces

¼ cup cucumber, peeled and diced into small uniform pieces

¼ cup carrots, peeled and chopped into small uniform cubes

1 tablespoon red onion, finely chopped

Fine grain sea salt and pepper to taste

¼ cup low-fat Greek yogurt

1 teaspoon fresh dill, chopped

½ teaspoon garlic, finely chopped

Fresh lemon juice (optional)

4 Boston or Bibb lettuce leaves (or romaine hearts), washed

¼ cup grape tomatoes, finely chopped

Preparation

1. If using raw chicken breast, heat olive oil in a skillet over medium-high heat until it shimmers, about 45 seconds. Add the chicken pieces and sauté until cooked through, about 5 minutes. Set aside on a plate and let cool to room temperature. (If using pre-cooked chicken, skip this step.)

2. When the chicken is at room temperature, combine it with the celery, cucumber, carrots, and red onion in a bowl. Season with salt and pepper and toss.

3. In a separate prep bowl, whisk together the Greek yogurt, dill, and garlic. Add salt and pepper to taste, and a squeeze of lemon juice, if desired. Stir well to combine.

4. Add the Greek yogurt dressing to the chicken salad and toss until all the ingredients are fully coated. Arrange the lettuce leaves on a plate and add one two heaping tablespoons of chicken salad to each leave. Serve immediately, or cover and refrigerate for a few hours until ready to eat.

Customizable Crostini

What I love about crostini is that you can personalize them in so many ways.
Depending on your appetite, time, and ingredients on hand, you can choose
your bread type, toppings, and how many you want to eat. If they are going to
be the entirety of my meal, for instance, I tend to have three. If I serve them as
a side with soup or salad, however, one or two is just fine. The basic principles
of preparation regardless of toppings are the same: pan-fry your bread in
olive oil; if using cheese, add it to the bread and melt it; sauté your vegetable
and add to your cheese toast. Then you can be creative with herbs and spices
to make your crostini work for your diet needs and palate. In other words, you
can't go wrong! Three variations I make often include broccoli with cheddar,
mushrooms and Gruyère, and plain sautéed zucchini with sea salt flakes.

Preparation Time: 10 minutes

Serves 1

Ingredients

2 tablespoons extra virgin olive oil, divided

1 slice healthy bread, ⅛-inch thick or to your liking (sourdough, whole grain, whole wheat, or sprouted are best)

1 to 2 ounces organic cheese, thinly sliced, shredded, or crumbled (cheddar, goat cheese, Manchego, mozzarella, Gruyère, ricotta, burrata, or vegan) (optional)

1 medium garlic clove, chopped

½ cup broccoli, mushrooms, and zucchini (or any vegetable of your choice, chopped into small pieces or cut into thin slices)

Fine grain sea salt and pepper to taste

Preparation

1. Heat 1 tablespoon of olive oil in a skillet over medium-high heat. Place the bread in the skillet and pan-fry both sides until just golden and crispy, about 2 minutes each side. Top the bread with cheese, if using a variety that warrants melting.* Reduce the heat to low and cover the skillet until the cheese melts, about 2 minutes. Once the cheese is melted, turn the heat off but leave the toast in the skillet to keep it warm while you prep your vegetable. (If you are not using cheese, or are using a variety that will be left uncooked, turn the heat off as soon as the bread is done pan-frying.)

2. In another pan over medium-high heat, add the remaining tablespoon of olive oil. Once the oil is shimmering, at about 45 seconds, add the garlic. Sauté the garlic until fragrant, about 30 seconds. Add your vegetable and sauté until tender (the time will depend on the vegetable).**

3. Plate the toast. Add your vegetable topping, salt and pepper to taste, and serve immediately.

*Certain cheeses such as Burrata and Ricotta are best uncooked. If using such cheeses, plate the bread before adding the cheese, and skip the melting step.

**Feel free to use condiments, herbs, and spices to add extra flavor to your vegetables. I like to throw in a bit of soy sauce to deepen the taste profile of my mushrooms. If you like heat, add a few red pepper flakes to your broccoli. Some fresh chopped basil turns burrata or mozzarella and tomato into caprese.

Zoodles with Pesto

A portmanteau of the words "zucchini" and "noodles," the zoodles trend hit hard and fast around 2017 and stuck: supermarkets from coast to coast now stock zoodles in their produce departments. Zoodles are perfect for a light, warm lunch and can even suffice for dinner, especially when combined with the potato cubes and green beans. The pesto recipe here is the same as the pesto on page 265, so if you have leftover sauce you can use it for those recipes, or vice versa. Note: be very careful when you are cooking the zoodles not to go past al dente, because otherwise they can taste off and have a mushy mouthfeel.

Preparation Time: 10 minutes

Serves 2

Ingredients

1 white potato, peeled and cut into small cubes about ¼-inch thick (optional)
1 cup string beans, cut into ¼-inch pieces (optional)
Fine grain sea salt to taste
2 tablespoons extra virgin olive oil
2 cups zoodles, or the equivalent amount of spiralized zucchini
1 recipe Liguria-Inspired Pesto (see page 265)
Pepper to taste

Preparation

1. If adding the potatoes and green beans: Bring a medium pot of water to a boil and add a pinch or two of salt. Add the potatoes and cook for about 5 minutes until they are tender but not cooked through. Add the greens beans to the pot with the potatoes and cook for an additional 5 minutes (the potatoes will cook for a total of 10 minutes and the beans for 5). When the potatoes and green beans are tender, drain and set aside.

2. Heat the olive oil in a skillet over medium-high heat until it shimmers. Add the zoodles and sauté, tossing continually with tongs for about 5 minutes, until tender but not soft. Add the pesto to the skillet and toss to coat them well. Salt and pepper to taste. If using, add the potatoes and string beans, tossing very lightly (so as not to disturb the potatoes) until evenly distributed. Serve immediately or let cool to room temperature, cover, and refrigerate until ready to eat.

Tofurky, Lettuce, Tomato, Avocado, and Cheese Sandwich

A traditional deli meat sandwich will no longer seem irreplaceable after you try this TLTAC. Unlike its counterparts, which are usually packed with calories, refined carbs, saturated fat, nitrates and nitrites, and sodium, this sandwich is a healthier choice that suits every eating pattern. If you need to take your sandwich on the go (car, plane, train, or hike), skip the avocado because once sliced, it will go bad very quickly. In addition, pack the Vegenaise in a separate container and spread it on your bread just before eating to prevent the bread from getting soggy.

Preparation Time: 5 minutes

Serves 1

Ingredients

2 thin slices whole grain bread
1 teaspoon Vegenaise
2 slices Tofurky
1 slice vegan cheese
2 tomato rounds, thinly sliced
¼ avocado, sliced into lengthwise ribbons
1 to 2 romaine lettuce leaves
Fine grain sea salt and pepper to taste

Preparation

Spread the Vegenaise on one slice of bread. On the other slice of bread, add the Tofurky, vegan cheese, tomato, avocado, and romaine, placing each ingredient neatly over the one below it. Season with salt and pepper. Close the sandwich and cut it in half. Serve immediately or pack in foil, plastic wrap, or a container, and store in the refrigerator until ready to eat.

Vegan Macro Bowl with Tahini Dressing

An intelligently designed mélange of vegetables perfectly sautéed and/or roasted makes for a filling lunch or dinner and a dish whose nutrition profile is hard to beat—thus the aptly named macro bowl, which refers to the balanced inclusion of all three macro-nutrients. For this recipe, I've chosen a random sample of colorful ingredients because the key is not exactly what you choose to include, but to "eat the rainbow," so you can pack in as many nutrients as possible. The sweet potato contains beta-carotene, vitamin C, and potassium as well as many other vitamins and minerals. The beets are a great source of fiber, folate, manganese, potassium, iron, vitamin C, and inorganic nitrates, which studies have shown can dilate blood vessels and reduce hypertension, as well as enhance athletic performance by reducing the body's need for oxygen. The chickpeas are full of protein, healthy carbohydrates, fiber, folate, iron, calcium, magnesium, phosphorous, and potassium. The yellow zucchini is a powerhouse of antioxidants such as carotenoids, zeaxanthin, and beta-carotene as well as many other vitamins and minerals (it's very robust in vitamin A). Finally, the broccolini is very rich in vitamins C and A, antioxidants, and fiber, while low in calories. But you can choose any combination of vegetables (think mushrooms, cauliflower, Brussels sprouts, kale) as long as they vary in color and draw from different families, such as cruciferous, root, and fungi. Have fun with it—you can experiment with this dish to your heart's content.

Preparation Time: 1 hour

Serves 2

Ingredients

3 tablespoons plus 1 teaspoon extra virgin olive oil, divided, plus more if needed

1 sweet potato, cut in half

4 small beets, washed and peeled

1 cup cooked chickpeas, either drained from a can or soaked overnight and cooked in water for 1 hour (or 90 minutes if needed) until tender

½ teaspoon cumin

½ teaspoon turmeric

Small pinch chipotle powder (optional or to taste)

1 cup yellow zucchini, chopped

1 cup broccolini, chopped

½ avocado, sliced lengthwise into thin ribbons

Fine grain sea salt to taste

Tahini Dressing (see page 266) to taste

Optional add-ins: tofu, tempeh, or seitan, pan-seared in olive oil, or any whole grain

Preparation

1. Preheat the oven to 400° F.

2. Pour a tablespoon of olive oil into a prep bowl and using a basting brush, brush the sweet potato halves with oil until thoroughly coated. Then wrap each half in aluminum foil and place on a sheet pan or in a Pyrex dish. Transfer the sheet or dish to the oven and roast the potatoes for 40 to 45 minutes, until tender all the way through. (Check by sticking a toothpick in their center.)

3. Place the beets on a sheet of aluminum foil. Using the basting brush, coat them evenly with olive oil (you can add more oil to the prep bowl if needed). Fold the foil into an airtight pouch around the beets. Place the beets in a Pyrex baking dish or on a sheet pan and transfer to the oven with the sweet potato. Roast the beets for 45 minutes, or until they are tender all the way through. (Test by taking the dish out of the oven, opening the foil pouch, and pricking the beets with a knife or toothpick.) When done, remove the beets from the oven and set aside to cool for about 5 minutes until they are cool enough to handle, but still warm. Then cut them into quarters.

4. Meanwhile, add the chickpeas to a small pot set over medium heat. Add a tablespoon of olive oil, the cumin, turmeric, and chipotle to the pot and stir to coat the chickpeas. Turn off the heat and cover to keep warm.

5. Heat a teaspoon of olive oil over medium-high heat until the oil shimmers. Add the yellow zucchini and sauté until golden, about 6 minutes total.

6. Heat the last tablespoon of olive oil in a pan over medium-high heat until it shimmers. Add the broccolini to the pan and sauté until just browned. Salt and pepper to taste. Set aside.

7. Using a large flat bowl, arrange the sweet potato, beets, chickpeas, zucchini, broccolini, and avocado side by side. Serve with tahini dressing drizzled on top or on the side as a dipping sauce.

Avocado Toast with Tempeh, Tomato, and Mustard Vegenaise

The beauty of avocado toast—and one of the reasons for this dish's ubiquitous popularity—is that it is completely customizable, from the type of bread used, to the preparation of the avocado, to the selection of ingredients on top. Eggs, Mexican street corn, kimchi, caprese, smoked salmon, radishes, and almonds are just a few of the creative choices I've seen. For this recipe, I've included tempeh, tomato, and mustard Vegenaise, and rather than do a traditional avocado smash, I slice the avocado, because slices have a less mushy mouthfeel and allow for a nice layering effect with the tempeh and tomato. The mustard Vegenaise spread adds a tangy note that complements the buttery avocado.

Preparation Time: 7 minutes
Serves 1

Ingredients

1 slice seven-grain, whole wheat, or sourdough toast
1 tablespoon Vegenaise (or another vegan mayonnaise of your choice)
1 teaspoon Dijon mustard
1 teaspoon extra virgin olive oil
3 to 4 thin slices tempeh
¼ avocado, thinly sliced into lengthwise ribbons
½ medium tomato, sliced into thin rounds from the bottom up to the stem
Fine sea salt and pepper to taste

Preparation

1. Lightly toast the bread in a toaster or on the stovetop. Set aside.

2. In a small bowl, combine the Vegenaise and mustard and mix until smooth. Set aside.

3. In a skillet over medium-high heat, heat the olive oil until it shimmers. Reduce heat to medium, add the tempeh slices, and sear them on both sides until golden, about 5 minutes.

4. Spread a thin layer of the mustard Vegenaise on the toast. Add the tempeh slices, followed by the avocado slices, and then the tomato slices. Salt and pepper to taste and serve immediately.

Roasted Sweet Potato with Sautéed Spinach and Cashew Cream

This recipe is a terrific lesson in meal planning and is perfect for lunch at home. Although the sweet potato takes a while to bake and the cashews need to soak overnight, both can be prepared in advance and will hold in refrigerator for several days. So, if you write this recipe into your meal plan for the week and dedicate some time for prepping, it's quick and easy to compose at mealtime. Once the cashews are soaked, the Cashew Cream only takes a minute to make, the spinach about 2 minutes to cook on the spot, and although the potato takes about 40 minutes to bake, you can work in the meantime. Covering all the macro-nutrients, a wide swath of micro-nutrients, antioxidants, and robust fiber, here you have a dish that is a major value-add to any diet in both taste and nutrition, and which will power you through a long afternoon of work or childcare, especially if you're not going to have time for a snack.

Preparation Time: 50 minutes

Serves 1

Ingredients

1 small to medium sweet potato, washed
3 teaspoons extra virgin olive oil, divided
Fine grain sea salt and pepper to taste
2 cups spinach, washed
1 recipe Cashew Cream (see page 268)

Preparation

1. Preheat the oven to 400°F.
2. Place the sweet potato in aluminum foil. Using a basting brush, brush a teaspoon of the oil to coat the potato evenly. Close the aluminum foil, pinching and folding the edges to make a pouch and transfer to a Pyrex dish. Place the Pyrex dish in the oven for 40 to 45 minutes, or until the sweet potato is soft all the way through. (Check by sticking the tip of a sharp knife or a toothpick in the center.)

(continued)

3. Heat a skillet over medium heat. Add the remaining teaspoons of olive oil and the spinach. Sauté the spinach until it's just wilted, about 2 minutes. Salt to taste.

4. Remove the potato from the oven. Open the foil pouch and slice the potato down the center. Let cool for about 2 minutes, then add the spinach between the potato halves. Drizzle the Cashew Cream over the spinach, season to taste with salt and pepper, and serve immediately.

Egg Salad with Mustard and Dill Vegenaise

Egg salad is protein-rich and contains vitamin B-12 and choline, among other important nutrients. It is also an extremely versatile dish you can easily serve on toast, in sandwiches, with healthy crackers, in salads, or simply on its own. Full of flavor thanks to the inclusion of mustard, fresh dill, and a nice amount of pepper, the taste of this recipe reminds me of deviled eggs, but it's far easier to make. If you recall from earlier in the book, studies recommend eating up to seven eggs per week, unless you have diabetes or high blood pressure, in which case, you should speak to your doctor and likely reduce to under three times per week.

Preparation Time: 15 minutes

Serves 1 to 2

Ingredients

2 eggs
2½ tablespoons Vegenaise
1 teaspoon Dijon mustard
1 teaspoon fresh dill, finely chopped
Finely ground sea salt and pepper to taste

Preparation

1. Bring a pot of water with the eggs to boil. Reduce the heat to medium and set a timer for 10 minutes. While the eggs are boiling, add a few ice cubes to a bowl of water. When the timer goes off, drain the eggs, then place them in the ice bath and refrigerate for at least 5 minutes. Remove the eggs from the ice bath and peel the shells.

2. Transfer the eggs to a separate bowl and mash them using the prongs of a fork (don't overmash; it's best to leave some small pieces of egg white and yolk for texture). Add the Vegenaise, mustard, dill, and salt and pepper. Mix well to combine the ingredients thoroughly. The final texture should be creamy but not completely smooth, with some small pieces of egg still intact. Serve with the accompaniments of your choice. The salad will hold in the refrigerator for up to 2 days.

Salads and Vegetarian Sides

Note: As illustrated in the meal plans (pp. 281–288), these dishes are usually paired with Lunch and Dinner Main dishes.

Raw Shaved Brussels Sprout Salad

Brussels sprouts are a quintessential fall and winter vegetable, which is when they abound on restaurant menus. A dish I love at a favorite neighborhood haunt, La Pecora Bianca, inspired this recipe. In my version, I've replaced sunflower seeds with walnuts and eliminated golden raisins, which are delicious but many don't care for. I've made up for the raisins with a dressing that includes maple syrup, whose sweetness similarly balances the sprouts' bitterness. Brussels sprouts are a cruciferous vegetable, which are important to incorporate into your diet on a regular basis. They contain a well-rounded group of vitamins including vitamins A, C, K, and folate. In addition, they contain bioactive compounds, which help prevent cell damage in the body. Though this recipe is written for one person, you can easily double it for two.

Preparation Time: 20 minutes

Serves 1

Ingredients

1 cup raw Brussels sprouts, washed and stem ends cut off
⅛ cup Parmesan, grated finely
1 tablespoon walnuts, crushed
1 small garlic clove, peeled
¼ teaspoon fresh lemon juice
1 tablespoon extra virgin olive oil
⅛ teaspoon maple syrup
Fine grain sea salt and pepper to taste

Preparation

1. Add the Brussels sprouts to a food processor with a slicing blade, then pulse the food processor until the sprouts are sliced very thin (if you don't have a slicing blade, you can use the S-blade and if you don't have a food processor at all, you can cut the sprouts very thinly on the vertical by hand). Transfer the shaved Brussels sprouts to a bowl. Add the Parmesan and walnuts and toss.

2. In a separate bowl, press the garlic. Add the lemon juice, olive oil, maple syrup, and a pinch of salt and pepper, then whisk until well combined. Pour the dressing over the salad and toss. Season with additional salt and pepper if needed. Serve immediately.

Flash-Fried Kale Salad with Eggplant and Walnuts

Although I'm a proponent of raw salads for lunch, not all stomachs can handle uncooked roughage, especially cruciferous vegetables like kale. This family of vegetables contains high levels of sulfur and fiber, which are hard to digest and can throw any system out of whack, particularly those with IBS, IBD, or Celiac. The good news is that some salads, like this one, are cooked and served warm and, because the kale is not cooked until wilted, the dish still has a leafy salad-like texture. Paired with hearty eggplant, the result is a sating meal with a good dose of calcium (about 55 milligrams per cup), as well as vitamins K, A, B-6, and C. Sometimes for an extra burst of color and flavor, I'll toss a couple of red grape tomato halves on the plate or top the eggplant with a few thin slices of roasted yellow peppers.

Preparation Time: 15 minutes
Serves 2

Ingredients

2 tablespoons extra virgin olive oil, plus 1 teaspoon,
    plus more for the eggplant if needed
1 small eggplant, sliced into thin rounds
4 heaping cups of Lacinato kale, washed, de-spined,
    and chopped into smaller leaves
1 tablespoon walnuts, chopped
High-quality aged balsamic vinegar for drizzling
Flaky sea salt and pepper to taste

Preparation

1. Add a tablespoon of olive oil to a prep bowl. Using a basting brush, liber-ally brush the eggplant rounds with the oil on both sides until thoroughly coated.

2. Heat a teaspoon of olive oil in skillet over medium-high heat until it shim-mers. Transfer the eggplant to the skillet and sauté on both sides, until soft, golden, and cooked through, about 5 minutes per side. As it cooks, press

(continued)

the eggplant down with a spatula to release the oil. If the eggplant appears dry (it should look shiny), add more oil to the pan. When done, transfer the eggplant to a plate lined with a paper towel (which will absorb some of the excess oil).

3. Using the same skillet, add the remaining tablespoon of olive oil and heat until it shimmers. Then, add the kale and flash fry it for about 45 seconds, tossing it continuously with tongs until it's partially but not totally wilted (it should still have a bouncy leaf-like quality). Remove the kale from the pan and plate it.

4. Arrange the eggplant on the kale, then sprinkle with walnuts. Add a drizzle of aged balsamic vinegar, the salt flakes, and pepper to taste. Serve immediately.

Burrata with Tomatoes, Roasted Bell Peppers, and Basil

When you're going to eat dairy, my theory is to make it worth it, and burrata is a great way to get your fill—I don't know a cheese lover who doesn't have a penchant for this decadent-tasting, creamy, tangy cheese. Paired with juicy ripe tomatoes, sweet roasted peppers, and aromatic basil, this salad isn't hard to make, but it's only as good as the quality of the ingredients. Burrata is best eaten close to the time it was made, and although you can find ripe tomatoes all year long, this dish excels in summer when tomatoes are at their peak.

Preparation Time: 20 minutes
Serves 2

Ingredients

1 yellow bell pepper, washed and cored
1 orange bell pepper, washed and cored
Extra virgin olive oil, for roasting the peppers, plus additional for drizzling
4 round slices medium or large ripe tomato
Fine grain sea salt and pepper to taste
1 2-ounce ball burrata, drained
Aged balsamic vinegar, for drizzling
1 teaspoon basil, chopped into ribbons

Preparation

1. Preheat the oven to 400°F.
2. Cut the peppers along their grooves, place them face-down on a sheet pan, and brush with olive oil so that they are completely coated. Transfer the sheet pan to the oven (or a toaster oven) and cook the peppers for about 25 to 30 minutes, until the skins are bubbling, loose, and charred. Remove the peppers from the oven and set aside until cool enough to handle. Carefully peel the skins off the peppers and cut them into about ⅛-inch-thick slices.
3. Place the tomato rounds on a serving plate and lightly season them with salt and pepper. Center the burrata on the tomatoes, then drape the roasted peppers over. Lightly drizzle the dish with olive oil and vinegar. Garnish with basil and serve immediately.

Summer Salad

This salad, inspired by the farm-fresh produce I enjoy during the summer on Long Island, is all about highlighting the flavor of the vegetables with high-quality, organic, cold-pressed extra virgin olive oil (something I recommend having on hand for many of the recipes in this book), lemon, basil, Maldon sea salt flakes, and pepper. It's a crowd-pleasing complement to antipasti, soups, and fresh bread.

Preparation Time: 5 minutes

Serves 1

Ingredients

1 mini cucumber, peeled and sliced into thin rounds (if not in season, use a regular one)

¼ cup cherry tomatoes, rinsed and cut in half (heirloom variety if possible)

1 ear corn, boiled until tender (about 4 minutes), then sliced from the cob to yield ¼ cup of kernels

⅓ avocado, cut into ½-inch pieces

2 teaspoons extra virgin olive oil

½ teaspoon fresh lemon juice

Flaky sea salt and pepper to taste

1 teaspoon basil or mint, chopped

Preparation

Add the cucumber, tomatoes, corn, and avocado to a small salad bowl. Drizzle the olive oil over. Add the lemon juice and salt and pepper to taste. Toss the salad and then garnish with basil. Serve immediately or cover with plastic wrap and refrigerate until ready to eat.

Baby Arugula Salad with Roasted Beets, Lentils, and Walnuts

Lentils are low in calories and a great source of protein, fiber, iron, folate, B vitamins, and polyphenols, which makes them a terrific toss-in to any vegetarian or vegan salad. Here I've combined them with arugula and roasted beets to get you well on your way to meeting your vegetable requirements for the day. Although some of the individual ingredients take time to prepare, you can cook the beets and lentils in advance (or purchase them pre-cooked) and store them in the refrigerator for up to a week.

Preparation Time: 1 hour (or 5 minutes if beets and lentils prepped in advance or bought ready to go)

Serves 1

Ingredients

2 small beets, washed and peeled
2 teaspoons extra virgin olive oil
Fine grain sea salt and pepper to taste
½ cup black, green, or brown lentils, canned or cooked from dried, rinsed, and picked over
1 heaping cup baby arugula, washed
6 walnuts, roughly chopped and lightly toasted
1 recipe White Balsamic Vinaigrette (see page 269)

Preparation

1. Place the beets on a sheet of aluminum foil. Using a basting brush, coat them evenly with olive oil. Season with salt and pepper and then fold the foil into an air-tight pouch around the beets. Place the beets in a Pyrex baking dish or onto a sheet pan and transfer to the oven. Roast for about 45 minutes, or until tender all the way through. (The cooking time will depend on the size of the beets; test by opening the foil pouch and pricking the beets with a knife or toothpick.) Remove the beets from the oven and set aside to cool to room temperature, then cut them into quarters.

(continued)

2. If using dried lentils, in a small pot set over medium-high heat, bring the lentils and 1½ cups water to a boil. Reduce the heat and simmer for about 20 minutes, until the lentils are tender. When done, strain and set the lentils aside to cool to room temperature, then add salt and pepper to taste. If using canned lentils, simply drain and rinse.

3. Plate the arugula, beets, and lentils side by side. Sprinkle the walnuts on top of the salad, drizzle or toss lightly with white balsamic vinaigrette, and salt and pepper to taste.

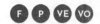

Go-To Lunch Salad with Hearts of Romaine, Cherry Tomatoes, Cucumber, Avocado, Walnuts, and Plant-Based Protein

Most people need a simple and quick lunch they can eat routinely, whether at home or on-the-job. This salad is easy to make and you can prepare the base ingredients in advance for three days at a time (save for the avocado, which needs to be sliced just prior to eating). If you have it several times a week like I do, you can create variety by switching the plant-based protein, the types of greens, and/or the dressing. If you have any leftover vegetables from dinner the night before, you can also toss those in. If you bring this salad to work, you'll want to keep it in the fridge until you eat it and consider eliminating the avocado, which doesn't keep well for very long after slicing.

Preparation Time: 10 minutes

Serves 1

Ingredients

1 cup romaine hearts, washed and chopped (or other leafy green of your choice)

¼ cup cherry tomatoes, halved

¼ cup cucumber, peeled and cut into thin rounds, or quartered

¼ avocado, peeled and pitted, and served whole or cut into ¼-inch slices (optional)

5 walnuts, crumbled

½ cup plant protein, such as tofu, tempeh, or seitan;* a legume (canned in water and drained or prepared from dried); fish, such as tuna, smoked salmon, white fish salad; or organic turkey slices or organic chicken

Any leftover roasted, sautéed, or grilled vegetables

White Balsamic Vinaigrette (see recipe on page 269) or Tahini Dressing (see recipe on page 266)

Fine grain sea salt and pepper to taste

*Tofu, tempeh, and seitan should be sliced into rectangles and pan seared over medium to high heat with olive oil in a saucepan until golden on both sides, then cut into cubes, or in the case of tempeh, rectangles.

(continued)

Preparation

In a wide, shallow bowl or a piece of Tupperware, arrange each ingredient side-by-side. If eating immediately, drizzle the dressing over the salad and add salt and pepper to taste. If taking to work, pack the dressing in a separate container and wait until just prior to eating to dress the salad.

Spinach Salad with Mushrooms and Melted Goat Cheese

When goat cheese is served as a warm round in a salad, it's often molded, breaded, and deep-fried. While delicious, the deep-frying technique is labor and ingredient intensive, and frankly, not that healthy. This salad simplifies the process by simply heating the cheese while preserving the tasty interplay between the warm ingredients and raw ones. It won't disappoint, even if you skip the goat cheese all together—spinach topped with warm mushrooms is pretty sublime in itself.

Preparation Time: 10 minutes
Serves 1

Ingredients

4 teaspoons extra virgin olive oil
1 cup shitake, white button, or maitakes mushrooms, sliced
8 toasted hazelnuts, halved or crushed
1 round goat cheese, sliced about ½ inch thick off a log
1½ cups spinach, washed
1 teaspoon aged balsamic vinegar
Fine grain sea salt and pepper to taste

Preparation

1. Preheat the oven (or toaster oven) to 325°F.

2. Heat 2 teaspoons of the olive oil in a skillet. Add the mushrooms and sauté until crispy on the outside but tender on the inside, about 5 minutes. Turn the heat off and leave the mushrooms in the skillet on the burner so they remain warm.

3. Meanwhile, place the hazelnuts on a pan and transfer to a toaster oven or oven. Bake until the hazelnuts are golden, about 3 minutes. Remove the nuts from the oven and set aside.

4. Place the goat cheese on the same pan used for the nuts and transfer to the oven. Cook until it just begins to melt, between 3 and 5 minutes (it should still hold most of its shape).

(continued)

5. Add the spinach to your salad plate or bowl. Add the mushrooms to the spinach, centering them on the greens. Scatter the hazelnuts around the salad. Add the melted goat cheese on top of the mushrooms. Dress the salad with a few drizzles of aged balsamic vinegar and remaining 2 teaspoons of olive oil. Add salt and pepper to taste and serve immediately.

Mixed Green Salad with Sundried Tomatoes, Green Olives, Red Radish, and Pine Nuts, with White Balsamic Vinaigrette

Everyone knows vegetables are good for their health. But did you know they are also good for your mood? According to a 2018 study in Frontiers in Psychology, consuming vegetables and fruit can alleviate depression, low self-esteem, loneliness, worry, anxiety, stress, and distress, and increase life satisfaction, happiness, self-efficacy, and overall well-being. I personally can attest to the fact that I don't feel nearly as good when I eat meals short on vegetables, which is why I make a small simple salad like this to accompany more protein- and carb-focused meal components.

Preparation Time: 5 minutes
Serves 1

Ingredients

1 cup mixed dark leafy greens of your choice, washed and spun dry
3 sundried tomatoes, sliced horizontally into slivers
4 green olives, halved
2 radishes, sliced into thin coins
1 tablespoon pine nuts
1 recipe White Balsamic Vinaigrette (see page 269)
Finely ground sea salt and pepper to taste

Preparation

Plate the greens. Add the radish slices, bell pepper, and toasted pine nuts. Add a couple of teaspoons of White Balsamic Vinaigrette, salt and pepper to taste, and toss the salad. Serve immediately.

Roasted Beets with Micro Greens, Walnuts, and Warm Brie Cheese

Many people presume they don't like beets, but I've found that it's not hard to transform beet haters into beet lovers when they are roasted. Why? Roasting brings out their natural sweetness and eliminates the slimy texture of canned beets and sour taste of pickled beets that many find unappealing. Beets are a powerful addition to a meal plan with a plethora of nutrients including fiber, folate, manganese, iron, vitamin C, and antioxidants (betalains).

Preparation Time: 1 hour

Serves 1

Ingredients

2 small beets, washed and peeled

Extra virgin olive oil, for drizzling and dressing

½ cup micro greens, frisée, arugula, or another green of your choice

1 to 2 ounces brie cheese, sliced into a rectangle (or substitute with goat cheese)

6 walnuts, crumbled

Aged balsamic vinegar, for dressing

Finely ground sea salt and pepper, to taste

Preparation

1. Preheat oven to 400°F.

2. Place the beets in aluminum foil and drizzle with olive oil, using a basting brush to coat each beet evenly. Fold the foil making an air-tight pouch around the beets. Transfer the pouch to a Pyrex baking dish or onto a sheet pan and place in the oven. Roast the beets for 45 minutes, or until they are tender all the way through (test by taking the dish out of the oven, opening the foil, and pricking with a toothpick). When done, remove the beets from the oven and the pouch, and let cool for about 5 minutes until they are cool enough to handle, but still warm.

3. Meanwhile, add the micro greens to a salad plate. Then, slice the beets into quarters and arrange them tightly in the center of the greens, like petals of a flower. Add the brie on top of the beets so that their warmth melts the cheese. Sprinkle the walnuts around plate. Dress with a drizzle of aged balsamic vinegar and olive oil and add salt and pepper to taste. Serve immediately.

Eggless Caesar Salad with Tempeh Bits

My daughter is a Caesar salad aficionado, but I've never been a fan of raw fare, whether eggs in a Caesar dressing or fish in sushi rolls. In addition to the fact that uncooked food can harbor pathogenic microbes like salmonella and listeria, the idea and mouthfeel has never appealed to me. At the same time, I do love the flavors of a traditional Caesar salad, so I came up with an eggless spin on this much-loved dish. (I've also replaced the anchovies that are traditionally used in the dressing with tamari, so it's vegetarian.) I've added the option of including smoky tempeh bits for flexitarians trying to reduce their bacon consumption and others seeking a more robust meal. I hope you enjoy it as much as we do—even my daughter is a huge fan!

Preparation Time: 5 to 7 minutes

Serves 1

Ingredients

6 to 8 heart of romaine hearts, washed
1 tablespoon extra virgin olive oil, plus 1 teaspoon for the tempeh (optional)
¼ cup lemon juice, freshly squeezed
2 teaspoons red wine vinegar
1 teaspoon tamari
1 teaspoon grated Parmesan (or vegan Parmesan), plus a few larger thin slices
1 medium garlic clove, pressed or finely chopped
3 to 4 smoked tempeh strips, cut into very small rectangular pieces (optional)
Finely ground sea salt and pepper to taste

Preparation

1. Plate the romaine spears. (If you prefer a chopped Caesar salad, you can chop the romaine first and then toss the leaves with the dressing.)

2. Combine 1 tablespoon of olive oil, lemon juice, red wine vinegar, tamari, grated Parmesan, and garlic in a prep bowl. Whisk until emulsified. Drizzle the dressing over the romaine and top with the slices of Parmesan.

3. Optional: Heat a skillet over medium-high heat with the extra teaspoon of olive oil. Add the tempeh and sauté until golden, about 4 minutes. Sprinkle the tempeh over the salad, salt and pepper to taste, and serve immediately.

Frisée Salad with Danish Blue Cheese and Toasted Hazelnuts

Blue cheese isn't for everyone but for those who enjoy stronger flavored cheeses, it's a great add-in to salads, especially when you want one that is simple and light. This recipe uses Danish blue cheese, which is the mildest of the blue cheese family. The combination of the intensely flavored crunchy nuts, the light, crisp frisée, and the creamy, robustly flavored cheese kicks this salad up to a whole new level of interest. If you're absolutely not a fan of blue cheese, try substituting with feta, a crumbly goat cheese, or a couple slices of brie on the side.

Preparation Time: 5 minutes

Serves 1

Ingredients

1 tablespoon hazelnuts
2 cups frisée lettuce, washed and spun dry
White Balsamic Vinaigrette (on page 269)
Fine grain sea salt and pepper to taste
1 to 2 ounces Danish blue cheese, crumbled (or feta, goat, or brie)

Preparation

1. Preheat the oven to 325°F.
2. When the oven is ready, add the hazelnuts and toast until fragrant and golden, about 3 to 5 minutes. (Watch to ensure they don't burn.) Set aside and let cool.
3. Add the frisée lettuce to a salad bowl followed by the hazelnuts and a table-spoon of dressing. Lightly toss the salad until ingredients are mixed. Salt and pepper to taste. Plate the salad, then sprinkle the blue cheese over the top. Serve immediately.

Butter Lettuce Salad with Tomatoes, Avocado, and Chickpeas

Butter lettuce is a mild lettuce that many people like because it lacks the bitterness and fibrous texture of darker leafy greens like kale and arugula. While darker greens are usually touted for their nutritional benefits, lighter greens are also vitamin and mineral-rich. Standout nutrients of butter lettuce include vitamins A, K, and C, calcium, and iron. The inclusion of tomatoes, avocado, and chickpeas in this recipe rounds out its health profile by bringing antioxidants, monounsaturated fat, and protein to the table. If you enjoy this lettuce, it's not only terrific for salads but also great for layering in sandwiches and wrapping (instead of tortillas) for other vegetables and proteins.

Preparation Time: 3 minutes

Serves 1

Ingredients

2 cups butter lettuce, washed
4 grape tomatoes, halved
¼ cup cooked chickpeas
½ avocado, cut into chunks
1 tablespoon red wine vinegar
2 tablespoons extra virgin olive oil
1 teaspoon Dijon mustard
1 teaspoon organic maple syrup
Fine grain sea salt and pepper to taste

Preparation

Plate the lettuce. Add the tomatoes, chickpeas, and avocado. In a prep bowl, combine the vinegar, olive oil, mustard, and maple syrup and whisk until emulsified. Dress the salad and salt and pepper to taste. Serve immediately.

Chickpea "Caponata"

Caponata is a Sicilian dish made from a base of eggplant, onions, celery, garlic, olive oil, and then customized with other ingredients depending on the cook. Having always loved caponata's flavor profile, I developed my own plant protein-rich version by replacing the eggplant with chickpeas. In addition to protein, the chickpeas are replete with fiber, resistant starch (starch that moves through the small intestine undigested and feeds the good bacteria in the colon), polyunsaturated fatty acids, and other vitamins and minerals, especially folate, iron, calcium, magnesium, phosphorous, and potassium. The tomatoes add to the nutrition profile of this dish with the antioxidant lycopene. Although caponata traditionally rests for a period of time (somewhere between 1 and 3 days) before it is served so that the eggplant can absorb all the flavors, this version can actually be served immediately.

Preparation Time: 10 minutes

Serves 2

Ingredients

2 teaspoons plus 1 tablespoon extra virgin olive oil, divided
1 medium garlic clove, chopped
½ cup onions, chopped
⅔ cup chickpeas (canned in water, or dried and pre-cooked in boiling water until tender, about 45 minutes)
½ cup jarred organic tomato sauce, smooth
Fine grain sea salt and pepper to taste

Preparation

In a medium skillet, heat two teaspoons of olive oil over medium-high heat until it shimmers. Add the garlic and sauté for thirty seconds. Add the onions and continue to sauté until they begin to caramelize, about 7 minutes. Add the chickpeas, tomato sauce, and the tablespoon of olive oil to the skillet. Cook for 5 minutes, stirring regularly. Salt and pepper to taste and serve immediately.

Simple Herb Roasted Carrots

Carrots are full of antioxidants, most importantly beta carotene, which can be converted into vitamin A. Beta carotene is critical for eye health and helps kill free radicals that damage our cells. Studies show that this powerful nutrient may reduce the risk of heart disease and cancer, among other health conditions. Simply roasted carrots tossed with herbs make for incredible sides to any main dinner dish.

Preparation Time: 40 minutes
Serves 1

Ingredients

4 heirloom carrots (or 4 regular carrots), trimmed and peeled
2 teaspoons extra virgin olive oil
Fine grain sea salt and pepper to taste
½ teaspoon fresh thyme leaves, chopped
½ teaspoon rosemary leaves, chopped

Preparation

1. Preheat the oven to 400°F.
2. Place the carrots in a Pyrex dish or on a baking sheet, drizzle with olive oil, and toss to coat. Season with sea salt and pepper and toss again. Sprinkle the thyme and rosemary over the carrots. Transfer to the oven and cook for about 40 minutes, until tender all the way through (check at the 30-minute mark by inserting a toothpick or thin knife into the center).

    Note: Though the cook times will be different, you can roast many vegetables just like this if you prefer, using just extra virgin olive oil, salt, and pepper, and/or with the addition of herbs and spices of your choice. Some include: asparagus, beets, turnips, parsnips, Brussels sprouts, cauliflower, broccoli, bell peppers, winter squash, mushrooms, eggplant, onions, green beans, and potatoes.

Crispy Brussels Sprouts

My ex-boyfriend loved fried Brussels sprouts; if we went to a restaurant and they were on the menu, no doubt he would order them. As a home cook who reaps great pleasure from making food for my loved ones, I devoted time to mastering the not-so-easy task of making perfect deep-fried sprouts for him: crispy leaves on the outside and perfectly cooked tender and moist hearts on the inside. The key to achieving this was using a copious amount of canola oil rather than my go-to extra virgin olive oil (strongly flavored oils can enhance the sprouts' bitter taste and overwhelm their flavor) and the slicing of the sprouts. (I experimented with whole, halved, and quartered before I hit on very thin slices.) The results of those two tweaks were Brussels sprouts that were perfectly golden and crispy but not charred. The dryness also disappeared, and the taste of the Brussels sprouts was no longer bitter. Brussels sprouts are an important vegetable to break out from time to time to help diversify a meal plan: as a member of the cruciferous vegetable family, which also includes broccoli, cauliflower, kale, cabbage, collard greens, and bok choy, they pack in vitamin C, soluble fiber, and numerous phytochemicals.

Preparation Time: 10 minutes

Serves 2 to 4

Ingredients

Canola oil, enough to fill the bottom of the pot by about ½ inch
2 cups Brussels sprouts, washed, de-stemmed,
    and sliced vertically very thin
Fine grain sea salt and pepper to taste

Preparation

Heat the canola oil in a pot with a lid over medium-high heat until it shimmers. When the oil is hot, add the Brussels sprouts. Cover the pot and fry the Brussels sprouts, tossing them every couple of minutes, and checking them regularly until crispy and golden, but still tender (they can burn easily). The total cooking time should be about 7 minutes. Salt and pepper to taste. Serve immediately.

Plant-Based Meatballs

The road to any plant-based diet requires gradually reducing the amount of meat you eat, and the frequency with which you eat it. While that may sound daunting to some, there's a silver lining: many popular dishes can be adapted to be meat-free without sacrificing taste or satiety, these meatballs included. Intimidated for years to try my hand at making them, I could not have been more thrilled than when I finally got around to developing this recipe for homemade vegetarian meatballs. Not only are they delicious and satisfying, they're also incredibly versatile, making them a valuable component to a meat-free diet. You can enjoy them on top of a mound of spaghetti, in a macro bowl, or as I often do, on their own, topped with tomato sauce or pesto and served alongside a soup or a salad. Note: in addition to being vegetarian, this dish can be made gluten-free by using gluten-free panko crumbs.

Preparation Time: 1 hour
Makes about 12 meatballs

Ingredients

⅓ cup quinoa, or bulgur, or a combination of both
    (when cooked they will yield about 1 cup)
⅔ cups water
2 teaspoons extra virgin olive oil, plus 4 tablespoons, divided,
    plus additional for brushing the baking sheet
½ cup onion, chopped
3 medium garlic cloves, chopped
2 cups eggplant, diced into 1-inch cubes
⅓ cup Parmesan cheese or vegan Parmesan cut from a block,
    and then diced into small square pieces, plus 2 tablespoons
    grated for garnishing
¼ cup parsley, chopped
½ cup panko or gluten-free panko crumbs
3 tablespoons of your favorite organic marinara sauce
    (mine is Rao's marinara)
1½ teaspoons Italian seasoning
1 teaspoon fine grain sea salt to taste
Pepper to taste

(continued)

Preparation

1. Preheat the oven to 375°F.

2. Line a baking sheet with parchment paper.

3. Add the quinoa and the water to a small pot and bring to a boil. Reduce to simmer, cover, and cook until the quinoa has sprouted, about 15 minutes. Salt to taste. Fluff with a fork and set aside.

4. Heat the 2 teaspoons of olive oil in a large skillet set over medium heat until it shimmers. Add the onion and sauté until tender and translucent, about 5 minutes. Add the garlic at about the 3-minute mark and continue to sauté the onions and garlic together for the last 2 minutes. Set aside in a prep bowl.

5. Using the same skillet, add 2 tablespoons of olive oil and eggplant. Sauté over medium heat until the eggplant is golden and tender throughout, about 8 minutes. Salt to taste.

6. To a large food processor, add the quinoa, onions, garlic, eggplant, Parmesan, parsley, panko crumbs, 3 tablespoons marinara sauce, Italian seasoning, salt, and pepper. Pulse until the ingredients are well combined. The texture should be almost smooth but not completely.

7. Using an ice cream scooper, spoon out the mixture (1 scoop per ball) and then roll it in your hands, gently making one round ball at a time (if you're too rough with it, they will collapse). Place each ball on the parchment-paper-lined baking sheet, then transfer to the oven and bake for about 22 minutes, checking at the 20-minute mark to make sure they're not getting overdone. When finished, remove the sheet from the oven and serve the veggie balls as desired, on top of pasta, as a side dish, or in a macro bowl.

Easy Cumin-Infused Black Beans

Whether prepared as a side for tacos, a salad, or a vegetable dish, black beans are great to have around when you need a quick, tasty dose of protein. If making them from scratch, you will have to leave time for soaking (a few hours or overnight) and cooking (about 40 minutes), but you can also make a delicious batch quickly, straight from the can like I do here.

Preparation Time: 20 minutes
Serves 2 to 3

Ingredients

1 can black beans, packed in water
1 teaspoon ground cumin, plus ½ teaspoon more for additional flavor
1 teaspoon extra virgin olive oil
½ teaspoon fine grain sea salt, plus additional if needed
Pinch chipotle powder (optional)

Preparation

Pour the can of black beans into a small pot and bring to a boil (for a less saucy texture if you're adding to salads, drain the water from the beans first). Add the cumin, olive oil, and salt, and stir to combine. Reduce heat to low, place a lid on the pot, and simmer the beans until saucy, stirring occasionally, about 15 minutes. Add additional salt to taste and a pinch of chipotle powder for heat, if using. Serve immediately or let cool to room temperature, cover, and refrigerate.

Guacamole

Guacamole can be tricky because it contains several ingredients that can be divisive: cilantro, raw onions, and raw tomatoes. This very simple guacamole, therefore, is designed to be crowd-pleasing. It pairs well with many dishes, and can be made fast with a few basic ingredients: avocado, garlic, lime, and sea salt. However, if you prefer including some of the other add-ins, by all means you can very simply incorporate them at the end.

Preparation Time: 5 minutes
Serves 2

Ingredients

1 avocado
1 medium garlic clove, finely chopped
Juice of ½ fresh lime
Fine grain sea salt to taste
Pepper
¼ cup onion, finely diced (optional)
2 tablespoons cilantro (optional)
¼ cup tomatoes, diced (optional)

Preparation

Cut your avocado in half and remove the pit. Using a spoon, scoop the avocado flesh out of its skin into a bowl. Add the garlic, lime, and sea salt to taste. Mash with a fork, to your preferred smoothness, leaving some chunks of avocado intact if desired. Add and stir in any of the optional ingredients. Salt more to taste if needed and pepper if desired. Serve immediately or cover with an airtight covering and refrigerate for up to 1 hour.

Sautéed Zucchini

Ingredients

1 tablespoon extra virgin olive oil
1 large (or 2 small) zucchini, washed and sliced into thin rounds
Fine grain sea salt and pepper to taste

Preparation

Heat a tablespoon of olive oil in a medium skillet over medium-high heat until it shimmers. Add the zucchini and sauté until both sides are browned, about 3 minutes on each side. Add salt and pepper to taste and serve immediately.

Pan-Fried Olive Oil French Fries

Ingredients

¼ cup extra virgin olive oil
1 russet potato, washed, peeled, and cut into rectangular sticks
    about ⅛ inch thick

Preparation

Add ¼ cup olive oil to a large skillet and heat over medium-high heat until it shimmers. Add the potato sticks and fry until all sides are golden and crisp, about ten minutes total, turning them with tongs. Transfer to a plate with a paper towel, which will absorb any excess oil, then salt to taste and serve immediately.

Soups

Light and Silky Vegan Sweet Corn Bisque

This recipe is comforting any time of year but really shines in late summer when corn is at its peak. Corn gets a bad reputation because much of what's grown in the US is genetically modified. That said, organic GMO-free corn, fresh when in season and frozen when not, is easily procurable at many grocery stores and farm stands as well as online. A vegan alternative to a cream-laden bisque, this recipe makes for a healthier but equally delightful and silky soup.

Preparation Time: 10 minutes

Serves 1 to 2

Ingredients

2 teaspoons extra virgin olive oil
1 medium garlic clove, chopped
¼ teaspoon fresh ginger, grated
1 cup organic corn, frozen or sliced from the cob
Fine grain sea salt to taste
1 cup vegetable broth or water
1 tablespoon Cashew Cream (see page 268)
½ teaspoon vegan butter
Pepper to taste

Preparation

1. In a medium pot set over medium-high heat, heat the olive oil until it shimmers. Reduce the heat to medium, add the garlic and ginger, and sauté until fragrant, about 30 seconds. Add the corn. Sauté until the kernels are tender, about 5 minutes. Salt to taste. Add the vegetable broth and simmer. Transfer all ingredients from the pot to a blender (or in batches if using a small blender). Purée the soup until light and very smooth. Add the Cashew Cream and butter and blend again until completely combined.

2. Return the soup to the pot over medium heat for a few minutes. Salt and pepper to taste. When the soup is warmed through, ladle it into bowls. You can also cool the soup to room temperature, cover, and store in an air-tight container for up to a week in the refrigerator and 3 months in the freezer.

No-Pasta Minestrone Soup

I love pasta and I love vegetable soup but the very soft texture noodles take on when steeped in broth has never won me over. This recipe takes all of the flavors of a classic Italian minestrone, minus the pasta. The result? A nutritional powerhouse of vegetables and legumes immersed in a flavorful broth enriched by a Parmesan rind.

Preparation Time: 40 minutes
Makes 4 bowls or 6 cups

Ingredients

3 tablespoons extra virgin olive oil
1 yellow onion, chopped
½ cup grape tomatoes, sliced in half
3 carrots, washed, peeled, and diced
1 cup broccoli, washed and chopped
2 cups kale, washed, de-spined, stemmed, and chopped
3 cups vegetable broth
1 cup cannellini beans, canned in water
1 Parmesan rind
1½ teaspoons fine grain sea salt
Pepper to taste
Grated Parmesan, for garnish

Preparation

1. Heat 2 tablespoons of olive oil in a pot set over medium-high heat until it shimmers. Add the onions, reduce the heat to medium, and sauté the onions until soft and translucent, about 5 minutes. Add the tomatoes, carrots, and broccoli. Cover the pot and continue to cook for about 7 minutes until the broccoli turns bright green and the carrots begin to soften.

2. Add the kale and sauté until the leaves have wilted. Next add the vegetable broth followed by the cannellini beans. Bring the soup to a boil, then reduce to a simmer. Add the Parmesan rind.

(continued)

3. Cover the pot and allow the soup to cook, about 10 minutes, stirring occasionally and adding more vegetable broth if it becomes too thick. (This is a brothy soup, not a stew.)

4. Then remove the Parmesan rind, stir, and salt and pepper to taste. Serve immediately with a garnish of grated Parmesan. You can also let the soup cool to room temperature, cover, and refrigerate for 4 to 5 days, or freeze for up to 3 months.

No-Cream Cream of Asparagus Soup

Like all of my vegetable soups, this recipe is made with just a few ingredients and can be prepared quickly. (Note: you can easily skip the Cashew Cream without compromising taste.) It fits all eating patterns from flexitarian to vegan and pairs well with salads, sandwiches, flatbreads, casseroles, and myriad other side dishes and main courses. The optional addition of white truffle oil—a flavorful finishing oil that can be found at specialty grocery stores and online—adds a special kick. Asparagus is low in calories yet replete with nutrients including vitamins A, C, K, B-6, thiamin, and potassium, among others, as well as folate and fiber.

Preparation Time: 20 minutes

Serves 2

Ingredients

2 teaspoons extra virgin olive oil
1 cup onion, chopped
1 cup asparagus, washed, trimmed, and chopped
1 cup vegetable broth
1 cup water
1 tablespoon Cashew Cream (optional; see page 268)
¼ teaspoon fine grain sea salt, plus more to taste
White truffle olive oil (optional)
Pepper to taste

Preparation

1. Heat a pot over medium heat with the olive oil until it shimmers. Add the onions and sauté, stirring constantly until the onions are soft and translucent, about 5 minutes. Add the asparagus and sauté until bright green and tender, about 7 minutes. Add the vegetable broth and water and bring to a simmer. Transfer the ingredients to a blender (in batches if using a small blender). Blend on low until the vegetables are roughly chopped. Then increase the speed to high and purée until completely smooth. Add the Cashew Cream and salt and continue to blend for a few seconds until well combined. Pour the soup back into the pot set over low heat.

(continued)

2. When the soup is warmed through, ladle it into bowls. If using, add a drizzle of white truffle oil, then a dash of pepper, if desired. Serve immediately. You can also let cool to room temperature, cover, and store in an airtight container in the refrigerator for up to a week, or in the freezer for up to 3 months.

Classic Lentil Soup

My mother's lentil soup was a mainstay of my childhood, to which this recipe pays homage with one big adaptation: it's vegetarian. Whereas her version included chicken broth and diced hot dog, my version uses vegetable broth and diced carrots. Rich in protein, iron, folate, and fiber while low in calories and fat, this soup is a terrific component of any meal plan. Even though lentils don't require soaking (in contrast to most dry legumes which do), if you tend to bloat or suffer from overall abdominal discomfort when you eat them, it's not a bad idea to do so, because soaking can make them easier to digest, thereby reducing gas.

Preparation Time: 20 minutes (if using canned lentils) to 1 hour (if using fresh lentils)

Serves 4

Ingredients

1 tablespoon extra virgin olive oil
1 onion, chopped
1 cup carrots, washed, peeled, and diced
2¼ cups vegetable broth, plus more if needed
1 can brown lentils, packed in water (or 1 cup dry lentils soaked for a few hours to overnight)
½ teaspoon finely ground sea salt, plus more to taste
Pepper to taste

Preparation

1. Heat a sauté pan over medium heat. Add the olive oil, onions, and carrots, and sauté until the onions become soft and translucent and the carrots tender, about 7 minutes. (Make sure the onions don't brown.)

2. Bring the vegetable broth and lentils to a boil in a medium pot. Reduce the heat to low and add the carrots, onions, and sea salt. Stir to combine. If using canned lentils, simmer for 10 minutes or until the carrots are soft. If using dry lentils, simmer for 20 to 25 minutes until both the lentils and carrots are soft. Salt and pepper to taste. Serve immediately, or cool, cover and store in the refrigerator for up to a week, or in the freezer for up to six months.

Roasted Butternut Squash Soup

Butternut squash is a perfect example of why it's best to eat vegetables in season. Seasonal vegetables are not only optimally tasty, but are also the most nutritious they'll be during their life cycle. Although available year-round, butternut squash is at its peak in fall and winter, which is why we usually associate a sweet, nutty-flavored, warming bowl of butternut squash soup with leaves falling off trees. Like many soups, the flavors continue to bloom as the soup sits, so it's an ideal make-ahead meal you can have throughout the week. The Cashew Cream is preferred for texture and taste but if you're in a rush, you can skip it and the soup will still be delicious. The same goes for the toasted seeds; raw is perfectly fine if you don't have time for toasting.

Preparation Time: 50 minutes

Makes 2 bowls or 4 cups

Ingredients

1 cup butternut squash, peeled and cut into 1-inch cubes
    (you can purchase butternut squash peeled and cubed
    at certain supermarkets)
2 tablespoons extra virgin olive oil
1 cup onion, chopped
2 cups vegetable broth
½ teaspoon fine grain sea salt, plus more to taste
1 teaspoon butter or vegan butter
1 teaspoon honey, or maple syrup if making vegan
2 tablespoons Cashew Cream (optional; see recipe on page 268)
1 teaspoon pumpkin or sunflower seeds, toasted about 4 minutes
    at 325°F, until golden

Preparation

1. Preheat the oven to 400°F.
2. Place the squash cubes in a Pyrex baking dish or on a sheet pan and brush with a tablespoon of the olive oil. Transfer to the oven and roast the squash until soft and tender, about 35 to 40 minutes (open the oven and toss the squash with a spatula at the 15-minute mark).

3. Meanwhile, heat the other tablespoon of olive oil in a medium pot over medium-high heat until it shimmers. Add the onions and sauté until soft and translucent, about 5 minutes.

4. Remove the squash from the oven and transfer to the pot with the onions. Add the vegetable broth and bring to a boil. Then reduce the heat and simmer for 5 minutes.

5. Transfer the soup from the pot to a blender (in batches if blender is small) and blend until smooth and creamy. Stop the blender to scrape down the sides with a spatula and add the salt, butter, honey, and Cashew Cream. Blend again, adding a little extra water if needed for a thinner consistency. When done blending, transfer the soup back to the pot and cook over medium heat for another 5 minutes. Serve the soup immediately, topped with the toasted seeds, or cover and transfer to the refrigerator for up to a week. You can also freeze this soup for up to 3 months.

Creamy Creamless Vegan Broccoli Soup

I can't count the number of times I've eyeballed broccoli and cheddar soup on restaurant menus only to resist the indulgence. And here's the thing: I don't believe in depriving myself of delicious food just to eat healthy. I only make that sacrifice when the quality of the healthier product is as good as the less-healthy version, and in the case of broccoli cheddar soup, I have a worthy substitution. This soup exemplifies the win-win of eating nutritiously without compromising taste. It's just as delicious, if not more so, than the prepared broccoli cheddar soups I used to love so much, and it's loaded with healthy ingredients to boot.

Preparation Time: 15 minutes

Serves 1 to 2

Ingredients

1 teaspoon extra virgin olive oil, plus 1 tablespoon
½ cup yellow onion, chopped
2 cups broccoli, florets and stems, cut into ½-inch pieces
1¼ cups vegetable broth, plus more if needed for a slightly thinner consistency
1 tablespoon butter or vegan butter
¼ teaspoon fine grain sea salt, plus more to taste
2 tablespoons Cashew Cream (optional; see page 268)
Pepper to taste

Preparation

1. Heat 1 teaspoon of olive oil in a pot over medium-high heat until it shimmers. Reduce the heat to medium, add the onion, and sauté until translucent, about 5 minutes. Add the broccoli, and drizzle the remaining tablespoon of olive oil over the broccoli, stirring to coat evenly. Cover and cook for about 3 minutes, tossing about every minute or so.

2. When the broccoli is bright green, remove the lid and add the vegetable broth. Then add the butter and salt and stir with a wooden spoon. Replace the lid and cook for about 5 minutes.

3. Transfer all of the ingredients from the pot to a blender (in batches if blender is small) and blend until smooth and creamy. Add the Cashew Cream, if desired, and blend again until thoroughly combined. Gradually add a up to a tablespoon more vegetable broth if the consistency appears too thick. Taste and adjust seasonings, adding salt and pepper if needed. Serve immediately or let cool, cover, and chill in the refrigerator until ready to use. You can also freeze this soup for up to 3 months.

Vegetarian French Onion Soup

French onion soup typically gets its complex, unami-packed flavor from beef broth. When I learned I could achieve a meat-like depth of beef broth using a vegetable broth flavored with caramelized onions and tomato paste, however, I was quick to try my hand at a vegetarian version, and it worked beautifully. (Some people also use mushroom broth to stand-in for the beef.) This soup is a great example of how as a vegetarian, you can still enjoy your favorite meat-based dishes.

Preparation Time: About 1 hour

Serves 2

Ingredients

1 tablespoon extra virgin olive oil
2 cups onions, sliced into lengthwise into thin slivers
2 slices baguette, about ¼-inch thick
1 tablespoon butter or vegan butter
1 cup vegetable broth
2 teaspoons tomato paste
½ teaspoon fine grain sea salt, plus more to taste
1 cup Emmental cheese, grated on the large holes of a box grater
A few grinds of pepper to taste
Special equipment: Oven-proof soup dishes

Preparation

1. Preheat the oven to 325°F.

2. Heat the olive oil in a skillet over medium-high heat until it shimmers. Reduce the heat to medium, add the onions, and sauté until caramelized, about 15 minutes. (The onions should be soft and a deep golden color.)

3. Meanwhile, spread a thin layer of butter on each baguette slice, then transfer to the oven and toast until crisp. When done, remove from oven and set aside to cool.

4. Bring the vegetable broth and 2 cups of water to a boil in a small saucepan. Add the tomato paste, salt, and pepper, and stir to combine.

5. Place the soup bowls onto a sheet pan. Add one slice of baguette to each bowl, then divide the onions between the two bowls, placing them on top of the bread. Add 1 cup of the broth to each bowl. Let sit for a minute to let the bread absorb the liquid. Add more broth if the liquid level descends (which it likely will have due to the bread absorbing the liquid); you want only a small amount of room at the top of each bowl for the layer of cheese. Then add half a cup of cheese to each bowl, covering the soup like a lid.

6. Transfer the bowls to the oven. Bake for about forty-five minutes until the cheese is melted and bubbling with golden dimples and edges. Remove from the oven and let cool for about 10 minutes, then serve immediately.

Dinner Mains

Sole Meunière with Sautéed Zucchini and Pan-Fried Olive Oil French Fries

Grey sole is hands-down my favorite fish and it's easy to make at home. If you're not already in the habit of eating fish or are sensitive to varieties that taste "fishy," sole is a great primer for the taste buds. It's white and flaky, very mild in taste, and, when prepared well, has a melt-in-your-mouth quality. Like all of the fish I eat, I buy my sole at local seafood shops, where I know the fishmongers who can tell me what is fresh and sustainably caught, as well as the sizes of the servings, which change frequently: one day a single piece can be so small it will leave you starving, while the next day's fillets can be overwhelmingly large. Given that people have different perspectives on what defines "small," "medium," and "large," it's helpful to know when speaking with your fishmonger how many fillets are equivalent to an appropriate serving size of fish, which for one person is about four ounces (recall the USDA recommendation of at least two servings of fish per week, totaling eight ounces). For a well-rounded meal, choose a non-starchy vegetable such as zucchini, spinach, collard greens, string beans, or broccoli as your first side dish, and pair it with virtually any style of potato or whole grain as a second side.

Preparation Time: 30 minutes

Serves 2

Ingredients

1 large (or 2 small) zucchini, washed and sliced into thin rounds

5 tablespoons extra virgin olive oil, divided, plus an additional ¼ cup for pan fries

1 russet potato, washed, peeled, and cut into rectangular sticks about ⅛ inch thick

All-purpose flour, for dredging

Fine grain sea salt and pepper to taste

2 5-ounce fillets of grey sole

2 tablespoons butter

1 tablespoon fresh lemon juice

1 tablespoon parsley, washed and chopped

2 thin lemon slices

Preparation

1. Preheat the oven to 225°F.

2. Heat a tablespoon of olive oil in a medium skillet over medium-high heat until it shimmers. Add the zucchini and sauté until both sides are browned, about 3 minutes on each side. Add salt and pepper to taste, then keep warm in an oven at 200°F or in the pan over very low heat.

3. Add ¼ cup olive oil to a large skillet and heat over medium-high heat until it shimmers. Add the potato sticks and fry until all sides are golden and crisp, about ten minutes total, turning them with tongs. Transfer to a plate with paper towel, which will absorb any excess oil, then salt to taste. Keep warm in an oven at 200°F or in the pan over very low heat.

4. Place the flour in a shallow bowl. Lightly salt and pepper the raw pieces of sole. Then dredge the fillets in flour, coating them evening on both sides. Shake off any excess flour.

5. Heat a large skillet over medium-high heat. Add half of the olive oil and half of the butter. When the butter begins to brown, add 1 fillet of the sole. (I don't recommend cooking more than 1 fillet at a time, so work in batches, dividing the cooking fats accordingly.) Cook the sole until it softens and becomes flaky, about 2 to 3 minutes per side. When the sole is on the second side, add half of the lemon juice to the pan and swirl. Transfer the finished fillet to a sheet pan and keep warm in the oven while you prepare the second one.

6. Once both fillets are cooked, transfer each to a plate with the Sautéed Zucchini and Pan-Fried Olive Oil French Fries. Pour any excess sauce in the pan over the fish, and garnish with parsley and a slice of lemon. Serve immediately.

Tofu Bowl with Charred Scallions Over Vanilla Infused Rice

As you've learned, my approach to healthy eating allows for consuming most foods, so long as it's in moderation. Although whole grains are the healthier choice with which to go on a regular basis, it's perfectly fine to enjoy white rice as an occasional treat. This recipe calls for white rice, because the delicate flavors of the vanilla would be lost if paired with a nuttier-tasting whole grain.

Preparation Time: 20 minutes

Serves 2

Ingredients

²/₃ cup white sushi rice
1¹/₃ cups water
2 vanilla beans
Fine grain sea salt to taste
1 tablespoon sesame oil, plus more if needed
1 loaf extra firm tofu, sliced horizontally into ⅛-inch rectangles
½ teaspoon extra virgin olive oil
6 scallions, cut the same size as the tofu rectangles
1 tablespoon hoisin sauce, or to taste (optional)

Preparation

1. Bring the rice and water to a boil in a small pot, then reduce heat to low. Cut the vanilla beans in half and scrape out the seeds, allowing them to fall into the rice. Discard the pods. Cover the pot and cook for about 15 minutes. When the rice has absorbed all the water, fluff it with a fork, and add sea salt to taste. Turn off your burner and cover the pot to keep the rice warm until ready to serve.

2. Meanwhile, heat the sesame oil over medium-high heat in a large skillet. When the oil shimmers, add the tofu. Cook the bottom side of the tofu until golden and crispy, about 5 minutes. Then flip and do the same for the second side, adding more sesame oil if needed.

3. In another sauté pan, heat the olive oil over medium heat. Add the scallions and sauté until they are slightly charred, about 3 minutes.

4. Divide the rice into two serving bowls. Arrange the tofu on the rice and garnish with the scallions. Drizzle hoisin sauce over each bowl of tofu and serve immediately.

Banza Penne with Liguria-Inspired Pesto

I'll never forget sitting atop a hill in Italy eating my first bowl of pasta with Ligurian pesto. Unlike the oily pesto I'd had at home, this pesto was creamy and the pasta dappled with small cubes of potatoes and green beans—a surprising and extremely palatable addition that changed my relationship with pesto forever. This recipe is an homage to that dish, but with high-protein Banza in place of regular pasta. (Whereas I still enjoy regular pasta when I eat at a restaurant, I prefer healthier alternatives when I make it at home. Banza, which is a brand of pasta made with chickpea flour, quickly rose to the top of my list. Available in a range of common pasta shapes, Banza noodles have a palatable mouthfeel when cooked correctly. However, Banza pastas fare even worse than traditional pasta when overcooked, so you need to watch the cooking times carefully and err on the side of al dente.) Banza works beautifully with the sauce because the chickpea flour used in it has a naturally high starch content, which when tossed with the oil of the pesto, emulsifies into a creamy sauce.

Preparation Time: 20 minutes

Serves 2

Ingredients

Fine grain sea salt to taste
1 russet potato, peeled and diced into small cubes
1 cup French green beans, washed, trimmed, and chopped
3 cups Banza penne
½ teaspoon olive oil
1 recipe Liguria-Inspired Pesto (see page 265)

Preparation

1. Bring a medium pot of water to a boil. Add a dash or two of salt. Add the potatoes and cook about 5 minutes, until tender but not cooked through. Add the green beans and cook for an additional 5 minutes. (The potatoes cook for a total of 10 minutes and the beans for only 5 minutes.) When the potatoes and green beans are tender, strain and set aside.

2. Bring a large pot of salted water to a boil. Add the Banza penne and cook for 5 minutes, until al dente, reducing the heat as needed to prevent the water from boiling over. At minute 5, strain the pasta over the sink reserving ½ cup of the pasta water. Set the pasta water aside.

3. Place the empty pot back on the stove over low heat. Drizzle some olive oil in the pot, enough to lightly coat its bottom. Add the penne followed by the pesto. Slowly add the pasta water, stirring as you do so, until the sauce becomes creamy (you likely won't need all the water). Then add the potatoes and green beans. Toss carefully to keep the potatoes intact, until the penne, potatoes, and green beans, are well coated with the pesto. (You may not use all the pesto.) Salt to taste, toss once more, then divide the pasta between two serving bowls. Garnish with additional grated Parmesan, if desired, and serve immediately.

Shrimp Scampi with Sautéed Broccolini and Millet

Shrimp is one of the three most frequently consumed types of seafood eaten in the United States, along with canned tuna and salmon. And that's a good thing, because it's high in protein and omega-3 fatty acids, as well as vitamins, minerals, and antioxidants. With just a few ingredients and steps, this recipe takes only about 10 minutes to make. Moreover, it pairs well with just about any sautéed vegetable and whole grain, which makes it easy for first-time cooks, those pressed for time, and those who need to make a meal out of whatever is in the pantry.

Preparation Time: 20 minutes
Serves 2

Ingredients

20 medium shrimp, cleaned
2 tablespoons extra virgin olive oil, plus additional for seasoning the shrimp
Fine grain sea salt and pepper to taste
⅔ cup millet
½ teaspoon coconut oil
1 cup broccolini, chopped
2 medium garlic cloves, chopped
2 tablespoons butter
1 tablespoon fresh lemon juice
1 tablespoon parsley, chopped

Preparation

1. Add the shrimp to a bowl and lightly coat with olive oil. Season with salt and pepper. Toss and set aside to marinate for a few minutes.

2. Add the millet to a pot with 1⅓ cups of water, bring to a boil, then reduce heat to low. Stir in the coconut oil, place a lid on the pot, and cook until the millet has absorbed all the water and sprouted, about 15 minutes. (Check the package for exact cooking time.) When the millet is done, remove the lid from the pot, fluff it with a fork, and salt to taste. If the millet seems too dry, add another tablespoon or two of water and cover until the water is absorbed. When done, salt to taste, cover, and turn off the burner to keep the millet warm while you prepare the broccolini and shrimp.

3. Meanwhile, in a separate skillet, heat 1 tablespoon of olive oil over medium-high heat. Add the broccolini and sauté until bright green and tender, with crispy floret tips, about 5 minutes. Salt to taste.

4. Add the second tablespoon of olive oil and garlic to another skillet set over medium-high heat and cook the garlic until fragrant, about 30 to 40 seconds. Transfer the garlic to a prep bowl. Reduce the heat to medium. Add the shrimp and cook for 3 minutes. Flip the shrimp with tongs and cook for another 3 minutes, until cooked through. Add back the garlic, then butter, and lemon juice and swirl the pan to coat the shrimp.

5. Divide the shrimp between two plates and pour any excess sauce from the pan over it. Garnish with the parsley. Serve immediately along with the millet and broccolini.

Saffron Risotto

Saffron is an ancient spice, historically used not only as a cooking ingredient but also for medicine and to dye clothes (thanks to its rich golden color). Due to its labor-intensive harvesting process (it takes more than 10,000 flowers to produce one ounce), it is the most expensive spice in the world by weight, but you need only a very tiny amount to achieve enough of its unique aromatic flavor to season a dish. (If you don't want to make the investment, you can also make this dish—a simple Parmesan risotto—without it.) When purchasing saffron, be sure to choose the threads rather than powder. Crushing the threads right before cooking will release the strongest, purest flavor; powdered saffron does not taste as fresh and can include additives.

Preparation Time: 30 minutes

Serves 2

Ingredients

2½ cups vegetable broth, plus ½ to 1 cup water if needed
1 pinch of saffron threads
1 tablespoon extra virgin olive oil
½ cup onion, chopped
¾ cup Arborio rice
¼ cup Parmesan cheese, finely grated
½ tablespoon butter
Salt and pepper to taste

Preparation

1. In a large pot, bring the vegetable broth to a simmer. Reduce heat to low to keep broth warm. Remove ¼ cup of broth from the pot. Crush the saffron into the divided broth and stir to release the flavor. Set aside. Pour the rest of the broth into a liquid measuring cup.

2. Heat olive oil in a large skillet over medium-high heat until it shimmers. Add the onion and season it with salt and pepper. Reduce heat to medium and sauté the onions until soft and translucent, about 5 minutes, stirring consistently. Add the Arborio rice and lightly toast for 1 minute, continuing

to stir so that it fully combines with the onions and doesn't overcook (you don't want the grains to turn golden). Add the saffron broth and stir with the rice. Then, pour the rest of the vegetable broth in, ½ cup at a time, stirring continuously, adding each successive ½ cup when the rice has absorbed the former. Cook until the risotto is saucy and the rice al dente, about 20 minutes. (If the consistency doesn't look creamy and the rice is still hard, add water very gradually and keep cooking until you get a thick sauce.)

3. To finish the risotto, add the Parmesan and butter and stir until well combined. Salt and pepper to taste, then divide the risotto between 2 plates, garnish with grated Parmesan, and serve immediately.

Pan-Seared Wild Salmon with Healthy Dill Sauce, Corn on the Cob, and French Green Beans

Whereas with many types of fish it can be difficult to distinguish between wild and farmed, when it comes to salmon, their differences can be palpable. Farmed salmon contains much more fat than wild, lending it a particular aesthetic, mouthfeel, and taste that doesn't suit every palate, which is why this recipe calls for wild. That said, if you prefer farmed salmon or that happens to be what's available, you can easily swap it in. With either type, you'll be fueling your body with healthy omega-3 fatty acids, which are critical for regulating blood flow (they initiate the release of hormones involved in blood clotting, contraction and relaxation of artery walls, and inflammation) and genetic functioning (they bind to receptors in cells that regulated gene expression and functioning), and thereby can be helpful in preventing heart disease, stroke, cancer, autoimmune disease, and other chronic illnesses. While dill sauce is often made with sour cream or regular mayonnaise, I've opted for Vegenaise, which is plant-based, has less saturated fat and cholesterol, and to me, tastes just as good.

Preparation Time: 20 minutes

Serves 2

Ingredients

½ cup Vegenaise (reduced fat if preferred)
1 tablespoon fresh lemon juice
2 tablespoons fresh dill, chopped
2 ears corn on the cob
1 teaspoon butter or vegan butter
Fine grain sea salt to taste
1 cup French green beans, washed and ends trimmed
2 teaspoons toasted sesame oil
1 medium garlic clove, chopped
Sprinkle or pinch sesame seeds
Pepper to taste
2 5-ounce wild salmon fillets (you can ask to remove the skin if you prefer)
2 teaspoons extra virgin olive oil

Preparation

1. In a prep bowl, whisk together the Vegenaise, lemon juice, and dill. Cover with plastic wrap and place in the refrigerator until ready to serve.

2. Bring a large pot of water to a boil. Add the corn and cook for about 4 minutes (to yield a crisp outer kernel and tender inner kernel). When done, remove the corn from the pot with tongs (or strain with a strainer). When the corn is cool enough to handle, rub with the butter, salt to taste, and set aside.

3. Bring a medium pot of water to a boil. Add the green beans, blanch them for 2 to 3 minutes, then strain and run cold water over them to stop the cooking.

4. Heat a medium skillet over medium-high heat. Add the toasted sesame oil, then add the garlic and cook until fragrant, about 30 seconds. Add the cooked green beans and toss until coated with the sesame oil and garlic. Sauté for about 5 minutes until the beans are tender but still have a slight crunch. Sprinkle sesame seeds on the beans. Salt and pepper to taste, cover, and turn off burner until ready to serve.

5. Lightly season the salmon fillets with salt and pepper. Heat the olive oil in a medium skillet over medium-high heat. When it shimmers, add the salmon. Cook until the bottom sides of the salmon develop a golden-brown crust, about 5 minutes. Flip and cook the second sides to achieve the same effect and until done to your liking. (For medium rare, 2 to 4 minutes; medium, 5 minutes; medium-well, 6 minutes; well-done, 10 minutes.)

6. Divide the salmon between 2 serving plates and top each fillet with a table-spoon of dill sauce. Plate the corn and green beans alongside the salmon and serve immediately.

Meatless Monday Stir Fry

An important component of maintaining a healthy and varied diet is to draw inspiration from different global cuisines. Too much of any one food type gets old and can lead to imbalanced nutrient intake. Yet cooking the foods of different cultures can be intimidating, because they require new or foreign ingredients that aren't in your repertoire. That said, many ingredients, such as spices and condiments, last for a long time, so once they are in your pantry, you'll have what you need to experiment further. This recipe requires several condiments common to Asian cuisines, and can elevate your cooking skills through learning how to cook with several different vegetables simultaneously. If the ingredient list looks daunting, don't worry; it's easy to adapt to whatever vegetables you have on hand. (Just remember that best results come from cooking each vegetable separately and then combining them rather than throwing them all in one pan.) It also pairs beautifully with any grain. Long grain brown rice is a great go-to, but a combination of red quinoa and bulgur is an interesting, less obvious coupling I also enjoy.

Preparation Time: 20 minutes

Serves 4

Ingredients

3 tablespoons sesame oil, divided
2 tablespoons low-sodium soy sauce
1 tablespoon tamari
1 teaspoon ginger, grated or finely chopped
1 medium garlic clove, peeled and chopped
2 tablespoons hoisin sauce
½ cup vegetable broth, room temperature, plus more if needed
1 block extra firm tofu, diced into cubes ½-inch thick
4 teaspoons extra virgin olive oil, divided, plus more if needed
1 carrot, peeled and cut into rounds ⅛-inch thick
1 cup canned baby corn, each stalk cut on the bias into thirds
1 small sweet yellow onion, peeled and sliced into thin lengthwise strips
1 cup mushrooms (shitakes or white preferred), washed and peeled
1 cup asparagus spears, bottoms trimmed and diced
2 heaping cups spinach, washed and spun dry
¼ cup raw cashews

Preparation

1. In a small mixing bowl, whisk together 2 tablespoons of the sesame oil, the soy sauce, tamari, ginger, garlic, hoisin sauce, and vegetable broth. Set aside.

2. Over medium-high heat, add the remaining tablespoon of sesame oil to a medium nonstick skillet. When the oil is shimmering, add the tofu cubes. Sear the tofu until golden and crispy on all sides (use tongs to rotate the cubes). Remove the tofu from the pan and set aside onto a piece of paper towel.

3. In the same pan, over medium heat, add 1 teaspoon of the olive oil. When the oil is hot, add the carrots and corn. Cook until the carrots and corn begin to soften, stirring occasionally, about 8 minutes. Add additional oil if needed. (The vegetables should glisten, not look dry.)

4. Meanwhile, heat another sauté pan over medium heat. Add the second teaspoon of olive oil. After about thirty seconds, when the oil is hot, add the onions. Sauté the onions, stirring consistently, until tender and translucent, about 5 minutes. Set the onions aside in a prep bowl.

5. In the same pan the onions were cooked in, add the last 2 teaspoons of olive oil followed by the mushrooms and asparagus. Sauté the mushrooms and asparagus, stirring occasionally, until tender and slightly golden, about 7 minutes. Add back the onions, and then the corn and carrots, and stir to combine all vegetables. Then add an additional drizzle of olive oil and the spinach. Cook until the spinach has wilted, about 1 minute. Add the tofu and cashews and mix again.

6. Pour the sauce into the sauté pan. Stir until all ingredients are thoroughly coated and the sauce thickens. Add more vegetable broth for a thinner consistency, if desired. Place a lid on the sauté pan and simmer for 3 minutes. Serve with a grain of choice or let cool and refrigerate for up to 3 days.

Lime Shrimp Tacos with Chipotle Crema

Taco Tuesdays is a much-loved tradition for people everywhere, regardless of diet, and preparations vary from traditional to fusion. This recipe is suitable for flexitarians and pescatarians, but the fact is you can fill a tortilla with whatever you want, so vegetarians and vegans should not feel left out. (See Vegetarian and Vegan meal plans for killer taco recipes suitable for those eating patterns.) These flavorful tacos are tangy and mildly spicy, light yet still filling. Importantly, when served with a side of cumin-infused black beans (recipe on page 195), it checks just about every nutritional box.

Preparation Time: 30 minutes

Serves 2 (makes 4 tacos)

Ingredients

¼ cup Vegenaise
¼ teaspoon ground chipotle, plus additional, if desired, for more heat
½ teaspoon Greek yogurt
½ teaspoon adobo sauce from a can of chipotle peppers (for heat; optional)
1 large tomato, washed
1 cup cabbage, washed and shredded
2 tablespoons extra virgin olive oil, divided, plus more for drizzling
¼ teaspoon fresh lemon juice
⅛ teaspoon organic maple syrup
Fine grain sea salt and pepper to taste
1 dozen medium shrimp, clean and de-veined
⅛ cup lime juice
1 medium garlic clove, chopped
4 organic small corn tortillas
1 recipe Guacamole (see page 196)
Cilantro, finely chopped
1 recipe Easy Cumin-Infused Black Beans (optional; see page 195)

Preparation

1. In a small bowl, stir the Vegenaise, chipotle, yogurt, and adobo sauce (if using) together until well combined. Set aside in the refrigerator until ready to use. Chop the tomato and set aside.

2. Add the cabbage to a medium bowl. In a separate prep bowl, whisk together 1 tablespoon of olive oil, the lemon juice, and the maple syrup. Add a pinch of salt and pepper. Pour the dressing over the cabbage and toss. Set aside.

3. Add the shrimp to another medium bowl. Add the second tablespoon of olive oil, the lime juice, and lightly season with salt and pepper. Toss and set aside.

4. Heat a medium skillet over medium heat. Add a drizzle of olive oil and the garlic. Cook the garlic until fragrant, about 30 seconds. Transfer to a prep bowl and set aside.

5. Add the shrimp to the same skillet in which you made the garlic and cook for about 3 minutes per side, until pink and cooked through. Cover the skillet and turn off the burner.

6. Heat another large skillet over medium-high heat. Drizzle a dime-size amount of olive oil in the pan for each tortilla and swirl to coat the bottom of the pan. Add the tortillas (two at a time if possible), and heat until warm on both sides but still soft and bendable (they should start to bubble as they warm up). Repeat until all four tortillas are warm.

7. Divide the tortillas between 2 plates. Add 3 shrimp to each tortilla. Top the shrimp with about a tablespoon each of cabbage and tomatoes. Garnish with the chipotle mayo, cilantro, and guacamole, and serve immediately with Easy Cumin-Infused Black Beans on the side if desired.

Chicken Paillard with Arugula Salad and Roasted New Potatoes

When I ate meat, chicken paillard was one of my favorite dishes. Pounded thin, pan-seared in olive oil, and topped with a lemony salad of arugula, tomatoes, and red onion, this dish is a tasty way to keep meat in your meal plan while avoiding red meat and some of its unhealthy accompaniments (gravies, casseroles, and thick sauces). What's more, if you are flexitarian and looking to improve the quality of your meat consumption, here's an opportunity to put your money where your mouth is. Buy 95 percent organic, pasture-raised chicken and master a cooking technique that requires neither deep-frying in animal fat nor the accompaniment of decadent, unhealthy sides.

Preparation Time: 40 minutes

Serves 2

Ingredients

2 cups new potatoes, washed and sliced in half, lengthwise
1 tablespoon extra virgin olive oil, plus more for drizzling
Fine grain sea salt to taste
2 sprigs rosemary, chopped
2 cups baby arugula, washed
⅓ cup grape tomatoes, cut in half
¼ small red onion, thinly sliced lengthwise
1 to 2 teaspoons fresh lemon juice
A drizzle of honey
2 3- to 4-ounce boneless, skinless chicken breasts,
    pounded flat to ¼-inch thick
¼ cup canola oil
Pepper to taste
1 tablespoon butter

Preparation

1. Preheat the oven to 400°F.

2. Place the potatoes in a Pyrex dish, drizzle with olive oil, and toss to coat evenly. Season with sea salt and rosemary, then transfer to the oven and roast for a total of about 45 minutes (Remove from the oven to toss at the 20-minute mark and check at the 35- and 40-minute marks to make sure they don't overcook. Precise cooking time will depend on the size of your batch of potatoes.)

3. While the potatoes are cooking, add the arugula, tomatoes, and red onion to a salad bowl. Lightly drizzle with olive oil, the lemon juice, and the honey. Salt and pepper to taste and toss again. Set aside.

4. Season both sides of the chicken breasts with salt and pepper. Add the canola oil to a large skillet. Heat the skillet over medium-high heat and, when the oil is hot, add the chicken breasts. Cook the chicken breasts for about 3 minutes, until the undersides are browned. (Jostle the pan every now and then to make sure they don't stick to the bottom.) Flip the breasts and do the same until the second side is browned and the chicken is cooked through, about 5 minutes. (You can test whether it is done by gently inserting the tip of a sharp knife into the breast; the knife should slide into the chicken easily and the chicken shouldn't feel fleshy or appear pink inside—it should be tender, moist, and white all the way through.) If needed, lower the heat to medium in order not to overcook the exterior of the chicken.

5. When the chicken is done, transfer it to a plate. Add the arugula salad on the chicken. Serve immediately with the roasted potatoes on the side.

Panko Crusted Sole with Sautéed Spinach and Wild Rice

Panko is a type of Japanese breadcrumb that is larger, flakier, and airier than most of its Western counterparts. (It is available in Asian markets, as well as many supermarkets.) There are two types of panko: white and tan. White panko is made with the white doughy part of bread only, whereas tan panko includes the crust. This recipe calls for white panko, which, when pan-fried, takes on the appealing golden and crunchy quality of deep-fried food. A question I'm frequently asked by those new to panko crumbs is whether they are they healthier than other breadcrumbs. The answer depends on the brand you buy, as some are more processed than others (avoid those with bleached wheat flour, added sugar, more than three to four ingredients, and added oil). That said, panko often has less sodium than regular breadcrumbs, and whereas regular breadcrumbs may have trans-fat, panko is usually trans-fat-free. If you're trying to move away from meat-based dishes like fried chicken and veal Milanese but are yearning for their crispy coating, this is a lighter and healthier way to satisfy your craving.

Preparation Time: 15 minutes

Serves 2

Ingredients

1 cup of wild rice
1 tablespoon butter, vegan butter, or coconut oil
Fine grain sea salt and pepper to taste
2 5-ounce fillets of sole
1 cup all-purpose flour
1 egg
1 cup white panko crumbs
2/3 cup extra virgin olive oil, divided
1 medium garlic clove, chopped
4 cups spinach, washed
4 very thin round lemon slices
1 tablespoon parsley, chopped

Preparation

1. Preheat the oven to 225°F.

2. Add the rice to a small pot with 2 cups of water and bring to a boil. Reduce the heat to low, add the butter or coconut oil, and place a lid on the pot. Cook for about 40 minutes, or according to the directions on the package. When the rice is done (plump and tender with all water absorbed), add salt to taste and fluff it with a fork. Turn the heat off but keep the pot covered on the burner to so that the rice remains warm while you prepare the fish and spinach.

3. Lightly season both sides of each fish fillet with salt and pepper. Place the flour in a shallow bowl. Crack the egg into a rectangular Pyrex dish (large enough to fit 1 fish fillet) and beat it. Spread the panko crumbs on a sheet pan. Dredge 1 sole fillet in the flour, shaking off any excess, then dip in the egg. When the surface area is completely coated with egg, place the fillet on the panko crumbs to coat both sides. Repeat with the second fillet.

4. Heat a large skillet over medium-high heat. Add 2 tablespoons of olive oil. When the oil is shimmering, transfer one fillet to the pan. Cook on one side until a golden crust forms, about 3 minutes. (The cooking time will vary depending on the thickness of the fish cuts.) With a spatula, carefully lift the fillet, add another 2 tablespoons of oil to the skillet, then flip the fillet and cook until the second side is golden, about another 3 minutes. When the first fillet is done, remove it from the pan and set aside on a large oven-proof plate with a paper towel on it. Dab the fish with the paper towel to absorb excess oil, then remove the paper towel and transfer the fish to the oven to keep warm while you cook the second fillet. (Even if the pan is large enough to cook both fillets at once, I find I get the best results by cooking them one at a time.) Add another 2 tablespoons of oil, then repeat the cooking method to pan-fry the second fillet, adding 2 more tablespoons of oil when you flip to the second side. When done, transfer the second fillet to the oven to keep warm while you cook the spinach.

5. In another large skillet heat 2 tablespoons of olive oil. Add the garlic and cook until fragrant and just golden at the edges, about 30 seconds. Add the spinach and sauté until wilted, about 1 minute. Salt and pepper to taste.

6. Remove the fish from the oven and divide the fillets between 2 serving plates. Garnish each fillet with 2 lemon slices and parsley. Add the spinach and wild rice on the side and serve immediately.

Baked Stuffed Sweet Potato with Cumin-Infused Black Beans, Melted Cheddar, and Greek Yogurt

Whether cubed and roasted, whipped, or baked and stuffed as in this recipe, sweet potatoes are a versatile ingredient. The key to this recipe is how the flavor from one ingredient (the cumin in the black beans) enhances the flavor of another (the inherent sweetness of the sweet potato). What's more, the cheese adds an indulgent-tasting gooey texture to the dish, which highly increases its satiety factor, while the cool Greek yogurt provides a pleasant contrast to the heated ones. What this dish is lacking in, however, is non-starchy vegetables, so I recommend serving it with a salad, vegetable soup, or sautéed vegetable on the side. Take it as a good rule of thumb to always pair any starchy dish with non-starchy vegetables.

Preparation Time: 45 minutes

Serves 1

Ingredients

1 small or medium sweet potato, washed
1 teaspoon olive oil
1 recipe Easy Cumin-Infused Black Beans (see page 195)
1 tablespoon white cheddar cheese (or vegan cheese), grated
1 tablespoon Greek yogurt (or vegan Greek yogurt)
Fine grain sea salt and pepper to taste

Preparation

1. Preheat the oven to 400°F.
2. Using a basting brush, coat the sweet potato with olive oil. Then wrap it in aluminum foil and place in a Pyrex dish. Transfer to the oven and cook the potato in its foil pouch for about 40 minutes, until knife tender. (Test by opening the foil pouch and pricking the potato to see that it is soft all the way through.)

3. Remove the potato from the oven and discard the foil pouch. When it is cool enough to handle, slice the potato halfway down the middle lengthwise, so both sides stay connected. Stuff the potato with 2 to 3 heaping tablespoons of black beans. Add the cheese on top of the beans. Let sit for about 2 minutes to allow the heat from the potato and beans to melt the cheese. Salt and pepper to taste, add the yogurt on top, and serve immediately.

Soba Noodles with Tofu and Vegetables in a Miso Broth

Cooking Japanese-style food is not my forte, but on occasion, when I'm feeling like a light vegetarian meal, I'll make soba noodles. Though soba noodles can be served warm or cold, I prefer them warm, whether steeped in a miso soup like in this recipe, or tossed in a heated sesame sauce and served like pasta. Soba noodles are a good example of how not all noodles are created equal. Healthier than white pasta, which is made with white refined flour, soba is made of 100 percent buckwheat. (Check the label when purchasing to make sure you are buying 100 hundred percent.) Buckwheat is an ancient whole grain, first cultivated more than 8,000 years ago, which is high in fiber, high-quality protein (with a strong amino acid profile), minerals, and B vitamins.

Preparation Time: 50 minutes

Serves 2

Ingredients

2 carrots, washed and peeled
2 teaspoons extra virgin olive oil
2 eggs (omit if vegan)
1 tablespoon sesame oil
½ block extra firm tofu, diced into ½-inch cubes
4 cups water
2 tablespoons red miso
¼ teaspoon fine grain sea salt
2 tablespoons tamari
2 scallions, thinly sliced on the bias
4 ounces soba noodles
2 cups spinach, washed

Preparation

1. Preheat the oven to 400°F.
2. Place the carrots in a Pyrex dish. Drizzle with olive oil, lightly season with salt, and toss until well coated. Transfer to the oven and roast for about 40 minutes, until the carrots are tender all the way through. Remove from oven and set aside. When cool enough to handle, using a sharp knife, slice the carrots into coins ⅛-inch thick.

3. Bring a medium pot of water to a boil. Add the eggs and cook them for 10 minutes, until hard boiled. When they are done, immediately strain the eggs over the sink and run them under cold water, then transfer them to an ice bath and refrigerate for 5 minutes. When ready, peel and slice the eggs in half, and set aside at room temperature.

4. Meanwhile, heat the sesame oil in a large skillet over medium-high heat until it shimmers. Add the tofu, and cook until lightly browned on all sides, about 5 minutes, turning the cubes with tongs. Turn the burner off while you prepare the miso broth.

5. Add 4 cups of water to a medium pot. Heat the water over medium-high heat until just before it boils. Add the red miso, sea salt, tamari, and scallions. Whisk until all the miso dissolves, then reduce heat to medium to keep warm while you prepare the noodles.

6. Bring a large pot of water to a rolling boil. Add the soba noodles and cook for about 4 minutes, or according to the packaging instructions until al dente. Strain the noodles over the sink and run cold water over them for about 20 seconds to remove any excess gluten. (The gluten will make the noodles sticky and cause them to clump.)

7. Transfer the noodles to the pot with the miso broth, then add the carrots, tofu, and raw spinach. Increase the heat to medium-high and cook until the spinach is wilted and the soup warmed through, about 3 minutes.

8. Using tongs, lift the noodles out of the soup and divide them between two bowls. Then, ladle the soup over the noodles, evenly distributing the vegetables. Add 2 egg halves to each bowl, yolks side up, and serve immediately. Salt to taste.

Tempeh Stir Fry with Spinach, Ginger, Garlic, and Soy Sauce

Stir fries are often thought of as "quick and easy," but this is not always the case; the amount of time it takes to make a stir fry actually depends on the ingredients it requires. For instance, some stir fries (such as the Meatless Monday Stir Fry on page 226) combine many vegetables, which each need to be chopped and have different cooking times and techniques. Slicing, dicing, and mincing the vegetables into unique cuts is time-consuming, as is measuring many seasonings and sauce ingredients. This recipe, however, takes stir frying down to its most accessible level, requiring only one plant-based protein, one vegetable, minimal seasoning, and just a single fat in which to cook everything. (It's also filling enough to eat on its own, though you can also pair it with a whole grain of your choice.) There's no doubt you can make it in a jiffy any night of the week. Leftovers also keep well for lunch the next day, or a meal later in the week.

Preparation Time: 15 minutes

Serves 2

Ingredients

2 teaspoons plus 2 tablespoons extra virgin olive oil, divided

2 medium garlic cloves, finely chopped

½ teaspoon fresh ginger, finely chopped

1 loaf tempeh, cut into ½-inch cubes

½ cup vegetable broth, plus a teaspoon or two more if needed

2 tablespoons low-sodium soy sauce

4 cups baby spinach, or another prepared vegetable of your choice
(snow peas cut horizontally into small rectangles, broccoli,
asparagus, peppers, onions, and mushrooms go very well too)

Preparation

1. Heat the 2 teaspoons of olive oil in a sauté pan over medium heat until it shimmers. Add the garlic and ginger and cook until fragrant, about 30 seconds. Remove the garlic and ginger from the pan and set aside in a prep bowl.

2. In the same pan, over medium-high heat, add the 2 tablespoons of olive oil. Add the tempeh and cook until all sides are golden (flip cubes with tongs as they crisp), about 3 minutes per side.

3. Once the tempeh is done, add the vegetable broth and soy sauce to the pan, followed by the spinach, garlic, and ginger. Stir well. Cover the pan with a lid and simmer for 5 minutes allowing the ingredients to absorb the flavors of the sauce. If too much liquid is absorbed (it should be saucy), add more broth, and, for a deeper flavor, feel free to drizzle in a bit more soy sauce.

4. Plate the stir fry and eat plain or with a whole grain of your choice. If you have leftovers, let cool, transfer to a container, cover, and refrigerate for up to 5 days.

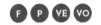

Middle Eastern-Inspired Stuffed Eggplant with Tomato and Cucumber Salad

It's always a bit stressful for me to test my vegan recipes on my omnivorous family and friends, but after several rounds of experimenting with variations of this dish, I finally introduced it to my mother and stepfather. I cooked everything at home in advance, including the pita, packed it up in the trunk of my car, and drove it over to their house. Happily, it was a huge success. Neither parent missed meat as the mainstay of their dinner. Note: if you're opposed tomatoes and eggplants because you've heard nightshades are bad for you, think again. Although they have some contraindications for folks with IBD, specific autoimmune diseases, or sensitivities and allergies to them, for most people, they can provide useful nutrients and can be part of a healthy diet.

Preparation Time: 45 minutes

Serves 2 to 4

Ingredients

2 large eggplants, washed, sliced in half, and scored
3 teaspoons extra virgin olive oil, divided, plus more for brushing eggplant
Fine grain sea salt and pepper to taste
1 cup cherry tomatoes, washed and sliced in half
1 cup cucumbers, peeled and chopped
2 scallions, chopped
1 teaspoon lemon juice
2 medium garlic cloves, chopped
½ cup walnuts, crushed
1 recipe Tahini Dressing (see page 266)
½ cup parsley, chopped
1 cup regular or vegan Greek yogurt

Preparation

1. Preheat the oven to 450°F.

2. Place the eggplant halves on a sheet pan, flesh side up, and brush them liberally with olive oil. Season lightly with salt and pepper. Transfer the pan to the oven and roast the eggplant for 30 to 35 minutes, until golden on top and tender all the way through. (Test by inserting a toothpick to make sure it's soft.) If the flesh is still tough, continue cooking. (Exact roasting time will depend on the size of your eggplants.) When the eggplant is done, remove it from the oven.

3. While the eggplant is cooking, in a small salad bowl, combine the tomatoes, cucumbers, and scallions. Add 2 teaspoons of olive oil, 1 teaspoon of lemon juice, and toss. Salt and pepper to taste and set aside.

4. Then, heat a small sauté pan over medium-high heat. Add the third tea-spoon of olive oil and sauté the garlic until fragrant, about 30 seconds. Set aside.

5. When the eggplant is ready, using a spoon, carefully scoop the eggplant meat away from the skins (trying not to tear them) and transfer to a bowl. Using a fork, smash the eggplant roughly, leaving some chunks. Add the sautéed garlic, walnuts, and a few drizzles of olive oil and mix well. Salt and pepper to taste. Using a spoon, transfer the eggplant mixture from the bowl back into to the skins. Top each eggplant half with a couple tablespoons of Tahini Dressing and tomato and cucumber salad. Add a dollop of yogurt and garnish with parsley. Serve immediately with warm pita on the side.

Fusilli with Creamy Mushroom Sauce

I've always loved creamy pasta dishes, but in the past, I rarely made or ordered them because, delicious as they are, I knew they weren't healthy. Enter Cashew Cream: a staple of vegan kitchens, it should, in my opinion, be a staple in any plant-based kitchen, as evidenced by how much I incorporate it into my recipes, and not just vegan ones. Cashew Cream provides the same texture as regular cream, but is healthier and not as heavy. Combined with NOOCH IT!, a seasoning that comprises nutritional yeast, organic cashews, organic brown rice flour, organic garlic powder, organic hemp seeds, and sea salt, you get the indulgent taste of fettucine alfredo, in vegan form.

Preparation Time: 20 minutes

Serves 2

Ingredients

Dash of sea salt, plus more to taste

2 cups whole wheat, chickpea, or fusilli pasta of your choice

4 teaspoons extra virgin olive oil, divided

½ cup yellow onion, chopped

1 cup white button or morel mushrooms (or another variety of your choice), stemmed and chopped into small pieces

1 cup vegetable broth

¼ cup Cashew Cream (see page 268), plus more if needed

1 tablespoon, plus 1 teaspoon NOOCH IT!

Pepper to taste

Preparation

1. Bring a large pot of lightly salted water to a rolling boil over high heat. Add the fusilli and cook according to the instructions on the pasta box minus 3 minutes, or just before al dente, then strain. (Do not rinse the pasta.)

2. Meanwhile, add a teaspoon of olive oil to a sauté pan set over medium-high heat. Add the onions and sauté until translucent, about 5 minutes. To the same pan, add the mushrooms and drizzle them with another teaspoon of olive oil. Sauté until the mushrooms are tender, about 7 minutes. Add the vegetable broth and Cashew Cream and stir until all ingredients are combined. Add the last 2 teaspoons of olive oil and stir. Add the NOOCH IT! Salt to taste, and stir again. Reduce heat to low and cover.

3. Add the pasta to the mushroom sauce and stir to coat. Cook until all the ingredients are warmed through, about 3 minutes. Salt and pepper to taste and serve immediately. If you have leftovers, let cool to room temperature, cover, and refrigerate for up to 2 days.

Seitan Piccata with Kale and Quinoa

Seitan is a plant-based protein made from wheat gluten (therefore not appropriate for Celiacs or anyone with a gluten sensitivity), the main protein in wheat. During the processing of seitan, the starch from the wheat is washed away, leaving only its protein. Whether you're flexitarian, pescatarian, vegetarian, or vegan, seitan can be very helpful when transitioning to a reduced-meat or meatless lifestyle. It has a unique flavor profile and its chewy texture allows it to act more like meat than tofu or tempeh. Whether in Asian-style stir fries, meatballs, chimichurri skewers, or lemony sauces like this one, seitan is highly versatile. (It also serves as the base for many processed vegetarian products such as vegetarian turkey, sausage, and bacon.) Although seitan lacks certain essential amino acids like lysine, it is high in protein, while low in carbohydrates and fat. As someone whose all-time favorite meat dish was veal piccata, this recipe fills a gap in my now-pescatarian diet. Quinoa, which is a complete protein (see page 86), and kale, which is very high in calcium and other vitamins and nutrients, round out this nutrient-rich meal.

Preparation Time: 20 minutes

Serves 2

Ingredients

1 cup quinoa
1 tablespoon coconut oil
Finely ground sea salt to taste
1 tablespoon extra virgin olive oil, plus 1 teaspoon
7½ ounces seitan, sliced into strips to yield about 1¼ cup
1 medium garlic clove, peeled and chopped
1 cup vegetable broth
1 tablespoon fresh lemon juice
1 tablespoon drained capers (optional)
¼ teaspoon maple syrup
1 tablespoon whole wheat flour
2 cups kale, washed, de-spined, and chopped (or baby kale, which does not
    require de-spining or chopping)

Preparation

1. Add the quinoa and 2 cups of water to a pot over high heat and bring to a boil. Reduce the heat to low, add the coconut oil, and place a lid on the pot. Cook the quinoa until sprouted, about 15 to 20 minutes. Remove the lid from the pot and fluff the quinoa with a fork. Salt to taste, turn the burner off, and put the lid back on the pot to keep the quinoa warm.

2. Meanwhile, heat the tablespoon of olive oil in a skillet over medium-high heat. Add the seitan and sear until golden with crispy edges, about 5 minutes. Reduce the heat and add the garlic, vegetable broth, lemon juice, capers (if using), maple syrup, whole wheat flour, and the additional teaspoon of olive oil. Cook, stirring constantly, until the sauce thickens and the seitan is thoroughly coated. Add the kale and stir until wilted. Check seasonings and salt to taste. (If the dish tastes too lemony, you can a little more maple syrup or vegetable broth to adjust.)

3. Plate the seitan and kale atop or beside the quinoa and serve immediately, or let cool and refrigerate for up to 4 days.

Tofu and Broccoli Curry

If you're not accustomed to using spices in general, this is a great place to start. The curry and turmeric flavors are light and subtle, and the spice is offset by the sweetness of the coconut milk. The result is a curry that is neither bracing nor too aromatic, which should be palatable to most taste buds.

Preparation Time: 40 minutes

Serves 4

Ingredients

1 tablespoon extra virgin olive oil
2 cups broccoli, rinsed and cut into florets
4 tablespoons water
2 tablespoons sesame oil
1 block extra firm tofu, cut into 1-inch cubes
1 cup full-fat coconut milk
1½ teaspoons curry powder, plus a dash or two more, if desired,
    for a more intense flavor
1 teaspoon turmeric powder
1½ teaspoons fine grain sea salt
Pepper to taste

Preparation

1. Heat the olive oil in a skillet over medium-high heat. Add the broccoli and stir to coat with the olive oil. Add the water. Then, with the florets face down, cover the skillet with a lid and cook for about 5 minutes, or until the water is full absorbed and the broccoli is bright green and tender with brown and crispy florets. (This technique of sautéing and steaming simultaneously allows the broccoli to both crisp and tenderize.)

2. In a separate pan, heat the sesame oil over medium-high heat. Add the tofu and cook until golden, rotating the cubes with tongs. When the tofu is done, add the broccoli (stir gently so as not to break or mash the tofu). Reduce the heat to medium. Add the coconut milk and stir to coat the broccoli and tofu. Add the curry, turmeric powder, and salt, and mix well into the sauce. Simmer for up 5 minutes, stirring occasionally. Salt and pepper to taste. Serve with a whole grain of choice. (My favorites are brown rice, bulgur, and millet.)

Spaghetti with Tomato Sauce and Plant-Based Meatballs

While it's okay to eat pasta made with white flour sometimes, there are innumerable variations on the market today made with healthier non-refined ingredients. From corn to whole wheat, brown rice to chickpea, quinoa to spelt flour, I'm sure you can find an alternative you enjoy more frequently. My favorites based on taste, texture, and how they hold sauces are corn, whole wheat, and Banza. While I give you the option to use any of these three in this recipe, feel free to use another one you prefer.

Preparation Time: 7 to 11 minutes
   (depending on what type of spaghetti you use)
Makes pasta for 2

Ingredients

Finely ground sea salt
5 ounces regular, corn-based, whole wheat spaghetti, or Banza
2 cups organic marinara sauce of your choice (I prefer Rao's)
1 tablespoon extra virgin olive oil
1 recipe plant-based meatballs

Preparation

1. Bring a deep pot of water and a dash of sea salt to a rolling boil. Add the pasta. Cook according to the packaging instructions minus 2 minutes, or until al dente. Drain the spaghetti over the sink. (Do not rinse.)

2. While the pasta is cooking, add the marinara sauce to a skillet over medium-high heat and stir. Then add the olive oil and stir to combine. Turn the heat to medium and keep the sauce warm until the spaghetti is ready.

3. When the pasta is done, strain and transfer it to the skillet with the sauce. Toss with tongs until the spaghetti is fully coated with the sauce. Salt to taste, then divide the spaghetti into two pasta bowls. Top with two or three plant-based meatballs and serve immediately.

Lemon Farro Risotto with Asparagus

Although I indulge in risotto made with the traditional Arborio or Carnaroli varieties of rice and Parmesan cheese from time to time, I devised this whole grain vegan version using the ancient Mediterranean grain farro as a risotto to consume on a more regular basis. (Farro's chewy texture and grain size make it a great substitution for Arborio and Carnaroli.) While those rice varieties are slightly refined, unpearled farro is not processed at all and is a great source of fiber, protein, iron, and magnesium. Since most farro in the United States is sold pearled or semi-pearled, check the package and buy whole, unpearled farro (or semi-pearled), if possible.

Preparation Time: 40 minutes

Serves 2 as a main course, or 4 as an appetizer

Ingredients

1½ cups water, plus a few additional tablespoons
1½ cups vegetable broth
1 cup farro (whole grain, if possible)
1 tablespoon extra virgin olive oil
1 cup asparagus, ends discarded and chopped into thin pieces,
    about ⅛-inch thick
Fine grain sea salt and pepper to taste
2 teaspoons vegan butter
½ tablespoon fresh lemon juice
¼ cup Cashew Cream (see recipe on page 268)
1 tablespoon NOOCH IT!, plus more for garnish

Preparation

1. Bring the water, vegetable broth, and farro to a boil. Reduce to a simmer and cover until the farro is tender. (Check the package because cooking time varies widely depending on the grain type; pearled takes about 15 minutes; semi-pearled about 30 minutes; whole grain about 40 minutes.) Stir every 7 to 10 minutes.

2. Meanwhile, heat the olive oil in a skillet set over medium heat, and sauté the asparagus until bright green and tender, about 5 minutes. Salt and pepper to taste.

3. Once the farro is tender, add the vegan butter, lemon juice, Cashew Cream, and asparagus to the pot. Simmer and stir occasionally for another 5 minutes adding more water if needed to create a creamier consistency. (The risotto should spread on the plate uniformly, not clump or separate from the sauce.) Add the NOOCH IT! and stir. Salt to taste. Divide the risotto between 2 serving plates, and garnish each with another dash of NOOCH IT! Serve immediately.

Tempeh Tacos

This recipe reminds me of the tacos I ate as a kid, even though the hard shells, ground beef, and toppings like shredded iceberg lettuce and pale tomatoes we had back then are no longer a part of my diet. The flavors of this dish, channeled through seasoned tempeh, vegetables, cheese, sour cream, and guacamole, are similar and even tastier than the ones of my memories. Having tested this recipe on meat eaters, many times, I guarantee you it's never a hard sell.

Preparation Time: 45 minutes

Serves 6 tacos

Ingredients

2 tablespoons extra virgin olive oil, divided, plus more for drizzling
1 cup tempeh, crumbled
1 cup asparagus, ends discarded and chopped into very small pieces
1 cup mushrooms (white button or shitake), chopped into very small pieces
½ cup organic marinara sauce
Pinch chipotle powder (optional, for heat)
6 medium corn tortillas (about 6 inches in diameter each)
6 tablespoons cheddar or vegan cheese, shredded
1 recipe Easy Cumin-Infused Black Beans (see page 195)
1 recipe Guacamole (optional; see page 196)
Sour cream or vegan sour cream (optional)

Preparation

1. Preheat the oven to 325°F.
2. Heat 1 tablespoon of olive oil in a large sauté pan set over medium-high heat. Add the tempeh and sauté until golden but still soft and tender. (Do not overcook; it should not be crisp.) Set aside.
3. In a separate medium pan, heat the other tablespoon of olive oil over medium-high heat. Add the asparagus and mushrooms and sauté until tender. (Add another drizzle of oil if the vegetables seem too dry.) Add the asparagus and mushrooms to the tempeh in the large pan. Reduce the heat to medium and add the tomato sauce. Stir the tempeh and vegetables until thoroughly combined and coated with the tomato sauce. Salt and pepper to taste, and add the pinch of chipotle powder, if using. Reduce the heat to low.

4. Place the tortillas on a baking sheet. Add 1 tablespoon of cheese to each tortilla. Transfer the tortillas to the oven and bake them until the cheese has melted but the tortillas are still soft, about 3 minutes. Remove the tortillas from the oven. (Alternatively, you can prepare the tortillas on the stovetop. A technique I like is to drizzle some olive oil in a pan and cook the tortillas until golden on both sides, but still soft. For this technique, sprinkle the cheese over after you cook the first side tortillas, then cover the pan with a lid to help the cheese melt).

5. Plate the tortillas and fill each with a heaping tablespoon of the tempeh, asparagus, and mushroom filling. Add a tablespoon each of black beans, guacamole, if using, and a dollop of sour cream. Salt and pepper to taste and serve immediately. The filling can also be stored in the refrigerator in an airtight container for up to 4 days.

Tofu Satay

When I was in graduate school in Los Angeles, my friends and I would break out of campus for lunch at our favorite Thai restaurant in Los Feliz. My routine order was a bowl of shrimp tom yum soup, sticky rice, and a side of peanut sauce. Although the peanut sauce was a great accompaniment to the rice, I still yearned to enjoy it like my meat-eating friends did, as part of a complete meal, lathered over a chicken satay. Later, when developing my recipes, I couldn't resist creating my own vegetarian (it's also vegan) satay with tofu instead of chicken. If you're unfamiliar with or still getting used to the taste of tofu, this recipe is a great one to try. Peanut sauce is a perfect complement to tofu, and its flavor really commands the dish. Serve with a whole grain of your choice for a more complete meal.

Preparation Time: 20 minutes

Serves 2

Ingredients

½ block extra-firm tofu
4 tablespoons sesame oil, divided
3½ tablespoons tamari, divided
2 tablespoons sherry vinegar or wine
2 medium garlic cloves, chopped
¾ cup full-fat coconut milk
½ cup unsalted peanut butter, smooth
1½ teaspoons curry powder
1½ tablespoons brown sugar
1 tablespoon lime juice
Pinch of cayenne pepper
Special equipment: Skewer sticks

Preparation

1. Pat the tofu with a paper towel to absorb as much of the water it was stored in as you can. Then cut it into 1-inch cubes and spear each cube onto skewer sticks (about 4 per stick).

2. For the marinade, add 2 tablespoons sesame oil, 2 tablespoons tamari, and the sherry vinegar to a prep bowl. Whisk until the ingredients are thoroughly combined. Pour the marinade into a Pyrex baking dish. Add the skewers and rotate them to coat all sides with the marinade. Set aside for 15 minutes.

3. Meanwhile, for the peanut sauce, add the garlic, coconut milk, peanut butter, curry powder, brown sugar, lime juice, 1 tablespoon sesame oil, 1½ tablespoons tamari, and cayenne to another prep bowl. Whisk the ingredients until well combined and smooth.

4. Once the tofu is ready, heat the remaining 1 tablespoon of sesame oil in a nonstick skillet over medium-high heat until it shimmers. Add the tofu skewers to the pan. Pan-fry the tofu until its skin is slightly golden, rotating the skewers so that the tofu cooks on all sides, about 3 minutes per side.

5. Transfer the skewers to a plate and drizzle with the peanut sauce. (Or if you prefer, serve the sauce on the side as a dipping sauce.)

Vegetarian Tacos

Being vegetarian doesn't mean you have to forfeit Taco Tuesdays and you don't need an animal protein to make tacos exciting. For many people the real draw of tacos are the toppings, like guacamole, salsa, and sour cream/Greek yogurt, all of which are vegetarian. And tortillas can showcase vegetables just as deliciously as they can meat. Though this recipe can work with pretty much any vegetable (such as broccoli, kale, spinach, lentils, sautéed onions, and peppers), here I've chosen to use caramelized eggplant and zucchini, a combination I love and make frequently.

Preparation Time: 10 minutes
Serves 2

Ingredients

1½ cups diced tomatoes
½ cup diced cucumbers
3 tablespoon extra virgin olive oil, divided, plus additional for drizzling
Finely ground sea salt and pepper
1 medium zucchini, sliced into very thin rounds
1 small eggplant, sliced into thin rounds
4 corn tortillas (5-inch)
⅔ cup organic Colby jack (or vegan) cheese, shredded
1 recipe Guacamole (see page 196)
Greek yogurt or vegan Greek yogurt (optional)
1 recipe Easy Cumin-Infused Black Beans (see page 195)

Preparation

1. In a prep bowl, combine the cucumbers and tomatoes. Toss with a drizzle or two of olive oil and salt and pepper to taste.

2. Heat 1 tablespoon of olive oil in a skillet set over medium-high heat until it shimmers. Add the zucchini and sauté until both sides are browned, about 8 minutes. Salt to taste. Remove from heat and set aside in a prep bowl. In the same skillet, add the remaining 2 tablespoons of olive oil and eggplant. Sauté the eggplant until golden and tender, about 10 to 12 minutes. If the eggplant appears dry at any point, add more oil (it also helps to press the eggplant with a spatula). Salt and pepper to taste and set aside in a prep bowl.

3. In the same skillet over medium heat, heat the tortillas on one side, then flip them. Reduce the heat to low and sprinkle some cheese on each tortilla. Cover the skillet and cook until the cheese melts, about 3 minutes.

4. Once the cheese has melted, uncover the skillet. Plate the tortillas and top each with a few slices of zucchini and eggplant, the cucumber and tomato salad, a tablespoon of guacamole, and a dollop of yogurt, if using. Salt and pepper to taste and serve immediately.

Vegetarian Power Buddha Bowl

As a vegetarian you could end up lacking in nutrients if you don't make a point of eating small amounts of eggs or dairy. (Blue Zone centenarians, for instance, are known to eat two to four eggs a week often as a side to a plant-based or whole grain dish.) It's therefore important to have a repertoire of dishes in your diet that can be enhanced by simply adding an egg, or dairy, or both, such as this bowl. Already full of vitamins, minerals, fiber, and antioxidants from the vegetables and chickpeas, adding an egg rounds the dish out with a complete protein, choline, vitamin B-12, and vitamin D, which are scarce, if present at all, in non-animal-sourced products.

Preparation Time: 40 minutes

Serves 2

Ingredients

4 heirloom carrots (or 4 regular carrots), trimmed and peeled
2 tablespoons extra virgin olive oil, divided, plus more if needed
Fine grain sea salt and pepper to taste
4 cups Lacinato kale, washed, de-spined, and chopped
1 cup chickpeas from a can, drained
½ teaspoon turmeric
½ teaspoon cumin, plus more if desired
1 large ear corn, shucked and washed, or 1 cup frozen corn kernels
2 teaspoons vegan butter, divided
Pinch of chipotle powder
1 egg
½ avocado, sliced lengthwise
1 recipe Tahini Dressing (see page 266)
Optional add-ins: tofu, tempeh, or seitan pan-seared in olive oil,
    or any cooked whole grain

Preparation

1. Preheat the oven to 400°F.

2. Place the carrots in a Pyrex dish or on a baking sheet, drizzle with one to two teaspoons of olive oil, and toss to coat. Season with sea salt and pepper and toss again. Transfer to the oven and cook for about 40 minutes, until tender all the way through. When done, set aside.

3. Heat 1 tablespoon of olive oil in a skillet set over medium-high heat until it shimmers. Add the kale and sauté until soft and wilted, about 5 to 7 minutes (add more olive oil if the kale seems dry). Salt and pepper to taste. Turn off the stove and cover the kale to keep warm until ready to serve.

4. Heat a teaspoon of olive oil in a small pot set over medium heat until it shimmers. Add the chickpeas and toss to coat them with the olive oil. Add the turmeric and cumin and toss again to coat the chickpeas with the spices. Salt to taste. Reduce the heat to medium and let the chickpeas sit until warm all the way through. Then, turn off the heat and cover the pot to keep warm until ready to serve.

5. If using an ear of corn, bring a large pot with water to a rolling boil. Transfer the corn to the boiling water, and then reduce the heat to medium. Cook for about 4 minutes, until the kernels are tender. Using tongs, remove the corn from the pot. When the cob is cool enough to handle, slice the kernels from the cob. Heat a skillet over medium-high heat and add the corn. (If using frozen corn, add the frozen corn directly from the package to the skillet—you do not need to thaw it.) Add one teaspoon of butter and salt and pepper to taste. Add the chipotle powder and sauté the corn for about 3 minutes.

6. Heat the remaining teaspoon of butter in a small skillet over medium heat. Crack the egg in the skillet. Fry to your liking—sunny side up or down, yolk soft or hard. (For a soft yolk, cook the egg for about 3 to 5 minutes; for a harder yolk, cook for about 7 to 10 minutes.)

7. In each of two large wide-bottomed bowls, arrange the kale, chickpeas, carrots, and corn side by side. Top the vegetables with the egg and avocado slices. Drizzle the Tahini Dressing over the dish, or serve on the side as a dipping sauce.

Frittata with Broccoli, Tomatoes, and Feta Cheese

Eggs for dinner often feels like a last-minute meal when there's no time to prepare anything else, but it doesn't have to be that way. An egg-based main course like a frittata with vegetables and cheese is a more creative endeavor that requires a little more time and focus. Here, I draw from the ingredients of a Greek salad to give the frittata a Mediterranean spin. For a lower-calorie, cholesterol, and saturated fat-free version, use egg whites instead of whole eggs. Serve with some roasted fingerling potatoes to make a complete meal that is delicious, filling, and thoughtfully put-together.

Preparation Time: 25 minutes
Serves 2

Ingredients

1 tablespoon extra virgin olive oil
1 cup broccoli, washed, de-stemmed, and chopped into small florets
1 tablespoon butter or vegan butter
4 eggs, beaten until light and fluffy (or egg whites)
Cherry tomatoes, washed and cut in half
⅓ cup feta cheese
1 tablespoon chopped basil, for garnishing (optional)

Preparation

1. Preheat the oven to 450°F.

2. Heat the olive oil in an 8- to 10-inch nonstick oven-proof skillet set over medium-high heat until it shimmers. Add the broccoli and sauté until tender and the floret tips are slightly crispy. Set aside in a prep bowl.

3. In the same pan, over medium heat, melt the butter. Add the eggs. As the bottom of the eggs begin to set, pull in their sides with a spatula and swirl the liquid to cover the pan again. Add the broccoli, tomatoes, and feta to the eggs, arranging them evenly to cover the full area of the pan.

4. Transfer the skillet to the oven. Bake until the eggs are fluffy and cooked through, 15 to 20 minutes. (Check the frittata at the 15-minute mark.) Add salt and pepper to taste. Slice the frittata into wedges (like slices of a pizza or cake), garnish with basil if desired, and serve immediately. You can also let cool to room temperature, cover, and store in the refrigerator for up to 2 days.

Whole Wheat Pizza 3 Ways

While a traditional Neapolitan pizza made with white flour is unbeatable in my opinion, this whole wheat take is a close second. Because the dough needs time to rise, I prefer to make this on weekends when I have ample time. (Bonus: use that time while the dough rises to experiment with toppings.) Plus, pizza night is a super-fun family activity in which kids love to partake.

Preparation Time: 2 hours
Serves 2 or 3 Small Personal Pizzas

THE DOUGH

Ingredients

1 envelope dry yeast
¾ to 1 cup warm water (between 105 and 115°F), plus more if needed
¾ tablespoon olive oil, plus additional for coating the bowl
2 cups whole wheat flour, plus more if needed
1 teaspoon sugar
¾ teaspoon fine grain salt

Preparation

1. Add the yeast to a small bowl. Add the warm water and whisk with the yeast. Set aside so that yeast can dissolve, about 5 minutes.

2. Meanwhile, brush a bowl with olive oil and set aside.

3. In another bowl or food processor, add and mix the flour, sugar, and salt. Then, add the yeast and water mixture to the dry ingredients, followed by the olive oil. If using a food processor, pulse a few times, gradually adding the water until a sticky ball forms, about 1 minute. If the dough is dry and doesn't form a ball, add more water until it does. If using your hands, on a floured surface, knead the dough for about 2 minutes until you get the same sticky ball. Mold the dough into a ball.

4. Transfer the dough to the lightly oiled bowl and turn it to coat with the oil. Cover the bowl with plastic wrap and set aside in a warm place for at least 1 hour so that it can rise. (For best results, let the dough sit for 3 to 4 hours.)

5. After the dough has risen to about twice its original size, punch it down. Cut the dough ball into 2 or 3 smaller balls, depending on what size and how many pizzas you want to make.

PIZZA MARGHERITA

Ingredients

⅓ cup thick tomato sauce (I like Rao's Marinara)
½ large ball fresh mozzarella, sliced into thin discs
Basil (optional)

Preparation

1. Preheat the oven to 425°F.
2. Roll out the balls of pizza dough into a very thin circle or oval. (I like my crust very thin, but you can leave it thicker if you prefer. And remember, they rise in the oven.) Transfer one ball to a baking sheet or pizza stone. With the back of a spoon, spread the tomato sauce around the pizza leaving ½ inch sauce-free at the edge of the dough for the crust to form. Place the mozzarella rounds on the sauce. Sprinkle the basil around the pizza. Transfer the pizza to the oven and cook for 10 to 12 minutes, checking at minute 10, until the cheese is bubbling and the dough is beginning to brown.

ZUCCHINI, FRESH MOZZARELLA, AND PARMESAN PIZZA

Ingredients

2 teaspoons extra virgin olive oil
1 medium zucchini, cut into thin coins about ⅛-inch thick
½ large ball fresh mozzarella, sliced into thin discs
1 tablespoon Parmesan, grated
Flaky sea salt to taste

Preparation

1. Preheat the oven to 425°F.
2. Heat the olive oil in a skillet over medium-high heat until it shimmers. Add the zucchini and sauté on both sides until golden, about 6 minutes total, 3 on each side. Transfer to a prep bowl.
3. Roll out a ball of the pizza dough into a thin circle or oval. (I like my crust very thin, but you can leave it thicker if you prefer.) Transfer the dough onto a baking sheet or pizza stone. Place the mozzarella on the dough. Arrange the zucchini coins on top of the mozzarella, followed by a dusting of Parmesan. Transfer the pizza to the oven and cook for 10 to 12 minutes, checking at minute 10, until the cheese is bubbling and the dough is beginning to brown. Remove from oven and garnish with a light dusting of sea salt crystals.

(continued)

MUSHROOM, MANCHEGO, AND CARAMELIZED ONION PIZZA

Ingredients

2 teaspoons extra virgin olive oil
1 cup mushrooms (of your choice)
1 medium yellow onion, sliced lengthwise into thin strips
⅓ cup Manchego cheese, shredded
Flaky sea salt to taste

Preparation

1. Preheat the oven to 425°F.

2. Heat one teaspoon of olive oil in skillet over medium-high heat until it shimmers. Add the mushrooms and sauté until tender. Transfer to a prep bowl. In the same pan, heat the remaining teaspoon of olive oil and add the onions. Sauté the onions until they caramelize, about 10 minutes.

3. Roll out a ball of the pizza dough into a thin circle or oval. (I like my crust very thin, but you can leave it thicker if you prefer.) Transfer the dough onto a baking sheet or pizza stone. Layer the mushrooms on top of the dough followed by the onions, and then the Manchego.

4. Transfer the pizza to the oven and cook for 10 to 12 minutes, checking at minute 10, until the cheese is bubbling and the dough is beginning to brown. Remove from oven and garnish it with a light dusting of sea salt crystals.

Banza Cacio e Pepe

It took me a while to find pastas I enjoy that are free of refined flour, but after some taste testing, I came away with a couple of very appealing options. Cacio e pepe, a pasta dish in which a long, thin pasta such as spaghetti is tossed in a mixture of black pepper and cheese, is one dish with which I've had great success using Banza. The starch from the pasta water combined with the Parmesan, olive oil, and butter make for a sauce just as creamy and delectable as one made with traditional white flour noodles.

Preparation Time: 10 minutes

Serves 2

Ingredients

6 ounces Banza spaghetti (or another white-flour-free pasta of your choice, such as whole wheat)
2 tablespoons extra virgin olive oil
1 cup Parmesan cheese, finely grated
1 cup pasta cooking water
2 teaspoons butter or vegan butter
Fine grain sea salt
1 teaspoon black pepper, plus more to taste

Preparation

1. Bring a large pot of water and a substantial pinch of salt to a rolling boil over high heat. Add the spaghetti. Cook for about 5 minutes (or 2 minutes less than the package says), then drain, reserving one cup of the pasta water.

2. Place the pot back on the stove over low heat. Add the olive oil and swirl it around the bottom of the pot. Then add the spaghetti back to the pot, and using tongs, toss the spaghetti to coat with the olive oil. Add the Parmesan cheese, then pour the pasta water over it so that it melts. Toss and stir the pasta again, until the cheese mixes well with the water to form a creamy sauce. Add the butter and toss again. Add a pinch or two of salt and then the pepper (if you are sensitive to pepper as I am, add it gradually and taste as you go along). Toss until the Parmesan has melted and is thoroughly combined with the pasta. Add additional salt and pepper to taste, and serve immediately.

Sauces
and Dressings

Liguria-Inspired Pesto

The region of Liguria, a crescent-shaped area along Italy's northwest coast known as "the Italian Riviera," is also the birthplace of pesto. When in season, basil grows in abundance there, and so pesto-making is a great regional pastime. The traditional Ligurian pesto technique requires grinding the basil with the other ingredients by mortar and pestle so that they combine as a smooth, creamy, and uniform sauce. Though here I forgo the mortar and pestle for the less time-intensive mini food processor, the result is surprisingly reminiscent of that pesto I had in Italy. If you're used to pesto that's a mess of oil and clumps of bitter basil like I was, you'll never go back. Note: in Liguria, and throughout Italy, pesto is made exclusively with Parmigiano-Reggiano, a specific type of Parmigiano cheese. For best results, seek out Parmigiano-Reggiano imported from Italy, rather than domestically produced Parmesan.

Preparation Time: 5 minutes
Makes ½ cup

Ingredients

¼ cup pine nuts
¼ cup basil
¼ cup Parmigiano-Reggiano (or Parmesan) cheese,
     plus additional grated cheese for garnish
2 tablespoons extra virgin olive oil
1 to 2 teaspoons water, if needed
Fine grain sea salt to taste

Preparation

Combine the pine nuts, basil, cheese, and olive oil in a very small blender or miniature food processor. Blend well, first on a low speed until the cheese is chopped finely, and then on a high speed until completely smooth. Pause to scrape the sides down as you go along, adding a little water if needed to achieve a smooth creamy texture. Add sea salt to taste, cover, and set aside until ready to use, or refrigerate for up to a week.

Tahini Dressing with Herbs and Spices

Tahini makes for a great dressing not only for veggie bowls, but also for salads when you're yearning for something other than vinaigrette. It is delicious plain with just lemon and salt, but can also be wonderfully flavored with spices and herbs. My favorite variation combines turmeric with cumin or curry powder. What's more, unlike many condiments, tahini is nutrient-rich and replete with protein (it has more than nuts), B vitamins, vitamin E, and several crucial minerals such as magnesium, iron, and calcium. This recipe yields a thicker, sauce-like consistency suited for macro bowls, but you can easily thin it out and transform it into a salad dressing by gradually adding a little more water and lemon juice.

Preparation Time: 5 minutes

Serves 2 to 4

Ingredients

⅓ cup tahini
⅓ cup water, plus more for a thinner consistency
1 teaspoon fresh lemon juice
¼ teaspoon fine grain sea salt and pepper to taste
Optional: ¼ teaspoon ground turmeric, ¼ teaspoon ground cumin, ¼ teaspoon curry powder, 2 teaspoons chopped parsley (feel free to combine more than one of these spices)

Preparation

Whisk the tahini and water together in a prep bowl until smooth. Add the lemon juice and whisk again until blended. Add salt and pepper to taste, followed by turmeric, cumin, and parsley, if desired. Whisk to combine. Set the Tahini Dressing aside for 5 minutes prior to serving. (It tends to thicken over time and might require more water after resting.)

Balsamic Vinaigrette

Although I tend to use white balsamic vinegar more frequently than dark (due to its subtle and clean flavor, I find it pairs better with most of the salads I eat), there are certain foods—caprese salad, sautéed bitter dark leafy greens like arugula, kale, and spinach, roasted root vegetables, and legumes—that thrive in the sweeter, syrupy, aged variety. The difference between white and dark balsamic vinegars has to do with how they are processed. Both vinegars are made from a white grape "must," which is a combination of the crushed fruit, seeds, skins, and stems. To make white balsamic vinegar, the must is pressure-cooked to prevent browning. It's then aged for only a short period of time yielding a clear, golden hue. For dark balsamic vinegar, however, the grape must is simmered for a very long time until it becomes syrupy and caramelized. Then it's aged for many years. A little bit goes a long way, adding both sweet and savory notes to the ingredients with which it is prepared.

Preparation Time: 3 minutes
Makes approximately ⅓ cup

Ingredients

¼ cup extra virgin olive oil
1½ tablespoons aged balsamic vinegar
1½ teaspoons Dijon mustard
1 medium garlic clove, chopped
Pinch fine grain sea salt
Pinch pepper

Preparation

Combine all of the ingredients together in a bowl and whisk until emulsified. Use immediately, or store at room temperature until ready to use. (If you double or triple the recipe to have on hand for subsequent meals, it can keep for up to a week or two in an airtight container in the refrigerator.)

Cashew Cream

Cashew Cream is a delicious vegan alternative to dairy cream you can add to various dishes from soups to vegetables to pasta and risotto. (I use it frequently in my cooking, as you'll notice from the number of times it appears in this book.) It's great for giving body to a dish as dairy cream would, but it can also be served as a dressing or sauce to finish. If you're using it as the latter, you can flavor it with spices and herbs of your choice. For spices, prepare the cream through the final step, then start with a quarter teaspoon of a ground spice like cumin, turmeric, or chipotle, whisk thoroughly into cream until blended, and increase the amount to taste, if desired. If using fresh herbs (parsley is one of my favorites), finely chop about a tablespoon of them, then mix into the finished cream. While this recipe requires a bit of prep time because the cashews need to be soaked for at least several hours to overnight, it comes together quickly and you can keep it in the fridge for up to a week.

Preparation Time: Several hours to overnight

Makes 1 cup

Ingredients

1 cup cashews, raw and unsalted, soaked overnight
2½ cups water, divided
⅛ teaspoon fine grain sea salt

Preparation

1. Add the cashews to a bowl with 2 cups of water. Cover and soak for 2 to 4 hours or overnight. (The longer you soak, the creamier and less cashew-tasting your cream will be).

2. After soaking, drain the cashews and transfer them to a blender. Add the remaining half cup water and salt and blend until the cream is silky and smooth. Depending on your usage, you can experiment with adding more or less water to achieve different consistencies.

White Balsamic Vinaigrette

*This is a dressing that suits any salad: flavorful but not overpowering. I like
to make enough of it (about four servings) at the beginning of the week to fill
a small Mason jar, since I eat my Go-To Lunch Salad almost daily. Because
the recipe calls for a three ingredients you might not regularly have on hand—
white balsamic vinegar, grainy mustard, and organic maple syrup—you
might need to make a trip to the market before you give it a shot. But the trip
is worthwhile because they are staples I recommended having on hand for this
recipe and others.*

Preparation Time: 3 minutes
Serves 2

Ingredients

¼ cup olive oil
1 tablespoon white balsamic vinegar
1 teaspoon grainy mustard
1 teaspoon organic pure maple syrup
Fine grain sea salt and pepper to taste

Preparation

Add all ingredients to a small bowl and whisk together until emulsified. Add
salt and pepper to taste. Serve immediately or cover and refrigerate until ready
to use.

White Wine Vinaigrette

Since many people are more likely to have white wine vinegar and Dijon mustard on hand than the ingredients my favorite dressing requires (see page 269)—white balsamic vinegar and grainy mustard—this is a classic French-style runner-up (without the commonly included shallots) that you can serve on any salad.

Preparation Time: 3 minutes

Serves 2

Ingredients

¼ cup olive oil
1 tablespoon white wine vinegar
1 teaspoon Dijon mustard
1 teaspoon organic pure maple syrup
Fine grain sea salt and pepper to taste

Preparation

Add all ingredients to a small bowl and whisk together until emulsified. Add salt and pepper to taste. Serve immediately or cover and refrigerate until ready to use.

Desserts

Moroccan Orange Salad

I'll never forget the orange tree-flanked streets of Marrakech, nor this incredible dish I found on practically every menu in that city. Though I learned that the trees, which line the streets there, bear oranges that are bitter and are solely for ornamentation, orange-infused food—couscous, tea, breads, desserts, lamb—from sweeter oranges still abounds. And I took full advantage of them. Throughout my trip, I ate salads like this one constantly as dessert. Though undeniably healthier than my typical dessert fare, the sweetness of the fruits combined with the nuts and spices made it feel just as indulgent, so much so that when I got home, I developed my own version. The beauty of this salad is that it's also great as a breakfast, side, or a snack, and of course is best when oranges are in season.

Preparation Time: 3 minutes

Serves 1

Ingredients

1 navel orange
2 dates, sliced into lengthwise slivers
1 tablespoon slivered almonds
Dash of cinnamon
Optional: Dollop of Greek yogurt (or vegan Greek yogurt)

Preparation

Cut off the top and bottom of the orange, then slice it into eights. Cut the center pulp off of each slice. Slide your knife beneath the orange flesh and slice the fruit away from its peel. Plate the orange slices, then top them with the dates, almonds, and sprinkle cinnamon over. Cover and refrigerate until ready to serve. (If adding the yogurt, do so just before serving.)

Vegan Chocolate Mousse

Traditional chocolate mousse always seemed like an out-of-reach delicacy to attempt in a home kitchen, until I learned that you could skip the most complicated steps and still yield great results by making it vegan. Here, there's no need for a double boiler to melt the chocolate, the hassle of perfectly separating and whipping eggs, or to concern yourself with constantly stirring. In fact, with just a few malleable ingredients, you can whip up this vegan chocolate mousse in just a few minutes. Note: the cashews must first be soaked for at least four hours to overnight.

Preparation Time: 5 minutes (plus 4 hours to overnight
    to soak the cashews)
Serves 2

Ingredients

1 cup cashews, soaked for at least 4 hours or overnight
½ cup water, plus more for a thinner consistency
2 tablespoons plant-based milk
1¼ tablespoons organic unsweetened cocoa powder
¼ teaspoon vanilla
1½ teaspoons maple syrup

Preparation

Add the cashews, water, and milk to a blender and blend until smooth. Add the cocoa powder, vanilla, and maple syrup and blend again. Cover and refrigerate for at least 15 minutes to chill before serving.

Vegan Nice Cream

Whenever I'm asked what my favorite food is, the answer is always ice cream. If I had to answer what my favorite flavor is, I would say coffee. But aside from pistachio and cherry, I'm not too hard to please when it comes to ice cream, which is why I like this recipe, which easily be adapted to whatever flavor I'm in the mood for. Admittedly, I have a weakness for Ben and Jerry's Chunky Monkey, which inspired the first recipe below. If you prefer a different flavor than banana, that mild taste can be easily transformed by the addition of other ingredients. Other favorites of mine include Chocolate Peanut Butter and Chocolate Raspberry.

Preparation Time: 5 minutes

Serves 2

THE NICE CREAM

Ingredients

2 frozen bananas
2 ice cubes, crushed
2 tablespoons almond milk (or another plant-based milk)

Preparation

Add the bananas, ice, and almond milk to a blender and blend until smooth and thick like frozen yogurt (do not over blend because the ice cream will lose its thick consistency). If adding flavorings, place the ingredients (see options below) in the blender with the nice cream and blend until completely combined but again, not over blended. Scoop the ice cream into a bowl and add toppings, if desired. Serve immediately.

FOR CHOCOLATE PEANUT BUTTER

Ingredients

2 tablespoons organic unsweetened cocoa powder
2 tablespoons of peanut butter
1 teaspoon pure organic maple syrup

Preparation

Add ingredients to the blender with the nice cream and blend until smooth and combined.

FOR CHOCOLATE RASPBERRY

Ingredients

2 tablespoons organic unsweetened cocoa powder
2 tablespoons organic raspberry jam
2 tablespoons organic almond butter
1teaspoon pure organic maple syrup

Preparation

Add ingredients to the blender with the nice cream and blend until smooth and combined.

FOR CHUNKY MONKEY

Ingredients

3 tablespoons coconut oil
1 cup chocolate chips
1 tablespoon chopped walnuts

Preparation

1. To make the Magic Shell: Add the coconut oil and chocolate chips to a bowl and microwave until melted, about 20 seconds. Remove from microwave and stir until well combined. If you see any remaining chocolate lumps, microwave again and stir more for a smooth consistency that drips in a thin stream right off your spoon.
2. Transfer the nice cream to two bowls, then add the walnuts and pour the Magic Shell over.

Vegan Vanilla Bean Rice Pudding

I've always loved creamy rice pudding with a hint of cinnamon, but as with all decadent desserts, I try to keep my consumption of it modest. Although this recipe is made with white rice, which is refined and not the healthiest food, it is otherwise fairly light; I've substituted the cream and/or milk with plant-based milk, and sugar for maple syrup. You can try swapping the white rice for a whole grain variety, but the results will not be quite as good.

Preparation Time: 30 minutes

Serves 4

Ingredients

2½ to 3 cups almond milk, plus more if needed (or another plant-based milk)
½ cup medium-grain white basmati rice
1 vanilla bean (you may substitute ½ teaspoon vanilla extract)
3 tablespoons maple syrup
1 tablespoon vegan butter
A pinch of salt
Optional: dash of cinnamon; berries; walnuts; chia seeds; flax seeds

Preparation

Add the almond milk and rice to a small pot set over medium heat and bring to a boil. Scrape the vanilla bean out of its pod and add to the mixture, followed by the pod itself. (Or vanilla extract, if using.) Reduce the heat to medium, bring the mixture to a simmer, and stir every few minutes to assist in the release of the rice starches and ensure that the rice doesn't stick to the bottom of the pot. When most of the milk is absorbed and the rice is tender (add more milk if it is not and the mixture is too clumpy), add the maple syrup, vegan butter, and salt. Stir to combine. Turn off the burner and pour the pudding into serving dishes. Allow the pudding to cool to room temperature and then chill for at least 30 minutes. Top with cinnamon or other toppings.

Vegan Chocolate Chip Cookies

Although I enjoy regular, non-vegan chocolate chip cookies from time to time, at home, I like to make this recipe, which can yield a soft, gooey cookie (as I prefer), or a crispier, crunchier one. While it does contain sugar, I've replaced butter with plant-based butter, all-purpose flour with whole wheat flour, and eggs with a flax seed and water alternative, all of which take it up a couple of notches from a nutrition perspective.

Preparation Time: 20 minutes
Yields about 14 medium sized cookies

Ingredients

1 tablespoon ground flax seeds
¼ cup warm water
1 stick plant-based butter, softened
¼ cup organic brown sugar
¼ cup organic white sugar
½ teaspoon vanilla
½ teaspoon salt
½ teaspoon baking soda
1 cup whole wheat flour
1 cup dairy-free semi-sweet chocolate chunks (or chips)

Preparation

1. Preheat the oven to 325°F.

2. Combine the flax seeds and water in a small prep bowl. Stir with a fork until blended. Set aside.

3. In a medium bowl, add the plant-based butter and sugars. Mix with an electric mixer until smooth. Add the flax seed and water mixture followed by the vanilla, salt, baking soda, and flour to this bowl. Mix again until thoroughly combined and smooth. Add the chocolate chunks and using a wooden spoon or spatula, fold them into the dough evenly.

(continued)

4. Spoon out the cookie dough and form each spoonful in ball 1 inch wide. Place the cookies on a baking sheet with about ¼-inch space between. Once all cookies are on the sheet, wet the spoon and gently flatten each cookie with the back of it.

5. Transfer the baking sheet to the oven. Bake for 8 to 10 minutes, until cookies reach your desired doneness. (For soft, gooey cookies remove at 8 minutes; for crispier cookies cook for 10 minutes.) Let the cookies cool a little, then serve either warm or at room temperature.

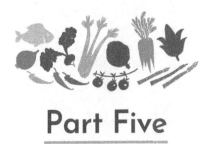

Part Five

SAMPLE MEAL PLANS

Flexitarian Meal Plan 1

Meal	Monday	Tuesday	Wednesday	Thursday	Friday	Saturday	Sunday
Breakfast	Fried Eggs with Turkey Sausage and Avocado	Steel-Cut Oatmeal with Cardamom, Cinnamon, Walnuts, and Maple Syrup	Morning Antioxidant Smoothie Vegan Thumbprint Corn Muffin	Homemade Granola with Milk and Berries	Morning Power Açai Bowl	Turkey Bacon, Spinach, and Cheddar Omelet 1 cup berries/fruit on the side	Guilt-Free Spelt Buttermilk Waffles with Maple Butter 1 cup berries/fruit on the side
Lunch	No-Cream Cream of Asparagus Soup Almond Flour Tortilla Flatbread	Go-To Lunch Salad with Hearts of Romaine, Cherry Tomatoes, Cucumber, Avocado, Walnuts, and Plant-Based Protein 1 slice Whole Wheat Zucchini Bread	Greek-Yogurt Chicken Salad in Lettuce Cups 1 slice Pan-Fried Sourdough Toast	Vegan Macro Bowl	Summer Salad Zoodles with Pesto	No-Cream Cream of Asparagus Soup Customizable Crostini	Go-To Lunch Salad with Hearts of Romaine, Cherry Tomatoes, Cucumber, Avocado, Walnuts, and Plant-Based Protein 1 slice Three Seed Bread
Snack	1 apple	¼–½ cup organic dried apricots	¼ cup dried chickpeas or fava beans	¼ cup raw unsalted nuts and/or seeds	1 piece or cup of fresh fruit	4 slices organic dried mango	¼ cup raw unsalted nuts and/or seeds
Dinner	Meatless Monday Stir Fry	Lime Shrimp Tacos with Chipotle Crema	Spaghetti with Tomato Sauce and Plant-Based Meatballs	Chicken Paillard with Arugula Salad and Roasted New Potatoes Simple Herb Roasted Carrots	Panko Crusted Sole with Sautéed Spinach and Wild Rice	Seitan Picatta with Kale and Quinoa	Soba Noodles with Tofu and Vegetables in a Miso Broth
Dessert	Moroccan Orange Salad	Vegan Vanilla Bean Rice Pudding	Vegan Chocolate Mousse	Vegan Chocolate Mousse	Vegan Chocolate Chip Cookies		Vegan Nice Cream

Flexitarian Meal Plan 2

Meal	Monday	Tuesday	Wednesday	Thursday	Friday	Saturday	Sunday
Breakfast	Vanilla Chia Seed Pudding with Cardamom 1 cup berries/fruit on the side	Egg White Frittata with Broccoli, Tomatoes, and Parmesan	Greek Yogurt Parfait	Poached Eggs with Pesto 1 cup berries/fruit on the side	Morning Antioxidant Smoothie topped with Homemade Granola	Whole Wheat Crepes 1 cup berries/fruit on the side	Whole Grain Almond Butter and Strawberry Jam Toast with Banana, Flax Seeds, Chia Seeds, and Walnuts
Lunch	Classic Lentil Soup Spinach Salad with Mushrooms and Melted Goat Cheese	Frisée Salad with Danish Blue Cheese and Toasted Hazelnuts Open-Faced Tuna Salad Toast	Classic Lentil Soup Baby Arugula Salad with Roasted Beets, Lentils, and Walnuts	Roasted Sweet Potato with Sautéed Spinach and Cashew Cream	Creamy Creamless Vegan Broccoli Soup Greek-Yogurt Chicken Salad in Lettuce Cups	Go-To Lunch Salad with Hearts of Romaine, Cherry Tomatoes, Cucumber, Avocado, Walnuts, and Plant-Based Protein. 1 slice Three Seed Bread	Egg Salad with Mustard and Dill Vegenaise 1 slice Pan-Fried Sourdough Toast
Snack	1 apple	¼–½ cup organic dried apricots	¼ cup dried chickpeas or fava beans	¼ cup raw unsalted nuts and/or seeds	1 piece or cup of fresh fruit	4 slices organic dried mango	¼ cup raw unsalted nuts and/or seeds
Dinner	Fusilli with Creamy Mushroom Sauce Sautéed Zucchini	Tempeh Tacos	Shrimp Scampi with Sautéed Broccolini and Millet	Chicken Paillard with Arugula Salad and Roasted New Potatoes	Vegetarian Power Buddha Bowl	Tofu Satay Simple Herb Roasted Carrots Crispy Brussels Sprouts	Pan-Seared Wild Salmon with Healthy Dill Sauce, Corn on the Cob, and French Green Beans
Dessert	Moroccan Orange Salad	Vegan Vanilla Bean Rice Pudding		Vegan Chocolate Mousse	Vegan Chocolate Chip Cookies		Vegan Nice Cream

Pescatarian Meal Plan 1

Meal	Monday	Tuesday	Wednesday	Thursday	Friday	Saturday	Sunday
Breakfast	Morning Anti-oxidant Smoothie 1 slice Whole Wheat Zucchini Bread	Scrambled Eggs with Avocado 1 cup berries/fruit on the side	Overnight Oats, Swiss Müesli Style	Bullseye 1 cup berries/fruit on the side	Morning Antioxidant Smoothie 1 slice Three Seed Bread	1 Vegan Thumbprint Corn Muffin 1 cup berries/fruit on the side	Fluffy Whole Wheat Vegan Pancakes with Maple Butter
Lunch	Go-To Lunch Salad Chickpea "Caponata"	Open-Faced Tuna Salad Toast Baby Arugula Salad with Roasted Beets, Lentils, and Walnuts	No-Pasta Minestrone Soup Raw Shaved Brussels Sprout Salad	Go-To Lunch Salad with Hearts of Romaine, Cherry Tomatoes, Cucumber, Avocado, Walnuts, and Plant-Based Protein	No-Pasta Minestrone Soup Egg Salad with Mustard and Dill Vegenaise	Flash-Fried Kale Salad with Eggplant and Walnuts Almond Flour Tortilla Flatbread	Burrata with Tomatoes, Roasted Bell Peppers, and Basil Summer Salad
Snack	¼ cup raw unsalted nuts and/or seeds	1 apple	4 ounces Vanilla Chia Seed Pudding with Cardamom	¼ cup raw unsalted nuts and/ or seeds	½ cup carrot sticks	4 slices organic dried mango	¼ cup raw unsalted nuts and/ or seeds
Dinner	Sole Meunière with Sautéed Zucchini and Pan-Fried Olive Oil French Fries	Vegetarian Tacos	Banza Penne with Liguria-Inspired Pesto Simple Herb Roasted Carrots	Mixed Green Salad with Sundried Tomatoes, Green Olives, Red Radish, and Pine Nuts, with White Balsamic Vinaigrette. Tofu Bowl with Charred Scallions Over Vanilla Infused Rice	Frisée Salad with Danish Blue Cheese and Toasted Hazelnuts Saffron Risotto	Pan-Seared Wild Salmon with Healthy Dill Sauce, Corn on the Cob, and French Green Beans	Vegetarian Power Buddha Bowl
Dessert	Vegan Nice Cream		Moroccan Orange Salad		Vegan Chocolate Chip Cookies		Vegan Chocolate Mousse

Pescatarian Meal Plan 2

Meal	Monday	Tuesday	Wednesday	Thursday	Friday	Saturday	Sunday
Breakfast	Morning Power Açaí Bowl	French-Style Omelet with Caramelized Onions, Mushrooms and Cheddar Cheese 1 cup berries/fruit on the side	Whole Grain and Almond Butter Strawberry Jam Toast with Banana, Flax Seeds, Chia Seeds, and Walnuts	Morning Antioxidant Smoothie 1 slice Three Seed Bread	Steel-Cut Oatmeal with Cardamom, Cinnamon, Walnuts, and Maple Syrup	Poached Eggs with Pesto	Guilt-Free Spelt Buttermilk Waffles with Maple Butter 1 cup berries/fruit on the side
Lunch	Creamy Creamless Vegan Broccoli Soup Avocado Toast with Tempeh, Tomato, and Mustard Vegenaise	Go-To Lunch Salad with Hearts of Romaine, Cherry Tomatoes, Cucumber, Avocado, Walnuts, and Plant-Based Protein 1 slice Three Seed Bread	Spinach Salad with Mushrooms and Melted Goat Cheese Plant-Based Meatballs	Go-To Lunch Salad with Hearts of Romaine, Cherry Tomatoes, Cucumber, Avocado, Walnuts, and Plant-Based Protein	Creamy Creamless Vegan Broccoli Soup Tofurky, Lettuce, Tomato, Avocado, and Cheese Sandwich	Mixed Green Salad with Sundried Tomatoes, Green Olives, Red Radish, and Pine Nuts, with White Balsamic Vinaigrette Roasted Sweet Potato with Sautéed Spinach and Cashew Cream	Roasted Beets with Micro Greens, Walnuts, and Warm Brie Cheese 1 slice Pan-Fried Sourdough Toast
Snack	¼ cup raw unsalted nuts and/ or seeds	1 apple	4 ounces Vanilla Chia Seed Pudding with Cardamom	¼ cup raw unsalted nuts and/ or seeds	½ cup carrot sticks	4 slices organic dried mango	¼ cup raw unsalted nuts and/ or seeds
Dinner	Tempeh Stir Fry with Spinach, Ginger, Garlic, and Soy Sauce	Lime Shrimp Tacos with Chipotle Crema	Fusilli with Creamy Mushroom Sauce Sautéed Zucchini	Vegetarian Macro Bowl with Cumin and Turmeric-Infused Chickpeas	Panko Crusted Sole with Sautéed Spinach and Wild Rice	Soba Noodles with Tofu and Vegetables in a Miso Broth	Whole Wheat Pizza 3 Ways
Dessert	Vegan Vanilla Bean Rice Pudding		Vegan Nice Cream		Vegan Vanilla Bean Rice Pudding		Vegan Chocolate Chip Cookies

Vegetarian Meal Plan 1

Meal	Monday	Tuesday	Wednesday	Thursday	Friday	Saturday	Sunday
Breakfast	Morning Antioxidant Smoothie 1 slice Three Seed Bread	French-Style Omelet with Caramelized Onions, Mushrooms, and Cheddar Cheese 1 cup berries/fruit on the side	Homemade Granola with Berries and Milk	Whole Wheat Crepes 1 cup berries/fruit on the side	Vanilla Chia Seed Pudding with Cardamom	Morning Power Açai Bowl	Egg White Frittata with Broccoli, Tomatoes, and Parmesan 1 cup berries/fruit on the side
Lunch	Roasted Butternut Squash Soup Almond Flour Tortilla Flatbread	Go-To Lunch Salad with Hearts of Romaine, Cherry Tomatoes, Cucumber, Avocado, Walnuts, and Plant-Based Protein 1 slice Three Seed Bread	Mixed Green Salad with Sundried Tomatoes, Green Olives, Red Radish, and Pine Nuts, with White Balsamic Vinaigrette Avocado Toast with Tempeh, Tomato, and Mustard Vegenaise	Spinach Salad with Mushrooms and Melted Goat Cheese 1 slice Three Seed Bread	Go-To Lunch Salad with Hearts of Romaine, Cherry Tomatoes, Cucumber, Avocado, Walnuts, and Plant-Based Protein. 1 slice Whole Wheat Zucchini Bread	Roasted Beets with Micro Greens, Walnuts, and Warm Brie Cheese 1 slice of Pan-Fried Sourdough Toast	Eggless Caesar Salad with Tempeh Bits Chickpea "Caponata"
Snack	¼ cup raw unsalted nuts	1 piece or cup fresh fruit	¼ cup organic dried apricots	¼ cup raw unsalted nuts	4 pieces organic dried mango	¼ cup dried chickpeas or fava beans	1 apple with almond butter
Dinner	Tofu Satay Crispy Brussels Sprouts	Vegetarian Tacos	Banza Cacio e Pepe Sautéed Zucchini	Vegetarian Power Buddha Bowl	Frisée Salad with Danish Blue Cheese and Toasted Hazelnuts Vegetarian French Onion Soup	Mixed Green Salad with Sundried Tomatoes, Green Olives, Red Radish, and Pine Nuts, with White Balsamic Vinaigrette Zoodles with Pesto Simple Herb Roasted Carrots	Whole Wheat Pizza 3 Ways
Dessert	Vegan Chocolate Chip Cookies		Vegan Nice Cream	Moroccan Orange Salad	Vegan Vanilla Bean Rice Pudding		Vegan Nice Cream

Vegetarian Meal Plan 2

Meal	Monday	Tuesday	Wednesday	Thursday	Friday	Saturday	Sunday
Breakfast	Morning Power Açai Bowl	Poached Eggs with Pesto 1 cup berries/fruit on the side	Overnight Oats, Swiss Müesli Style 1 cup berries/fruit on the side	Morning Antioxidant Smoothie topped with Homemade Granola	Vegan Thumbprint Corn Muffin 1 cup berries/fruit on the side	Guilt-Free Spelt Buttermilk Waffles with Maple Butter 1 cup berries/fruit on the side	Morning Power Açai Bowl
Lunch	Go-To Lunch Salad 1 slice Whole Wheat Zucchini Bread	Baby Arugula Salad with Roasted Beets, Lentils, and Walnuts Plant-Based Meatballs	Raw Shaved Brussels Sprout Salad 1 slice Three Seed Bread	Go-To Lunch Salad with Hearts of Romaine, Cherry Tomatoes, Cucumber, Avocado, Walnuts, and Plant-Based Protein. 1 slice Three Seed Bread	No-Pasta Minestrone Soup Tofurkey, Lettuce, Tomato, Avocado, and Cheese Sandwich	Burrata with Tomatoes, Roasted Bell Peppers, and Basil 1 slice Pan-Fried Sourdough Toast	No-Pasta Minestrone Soup Egg Salad with Mustard and Dill Vegenaise
Snack	1 apple	¼–½ cup organic dried apricots	¼ cup dried chickpeas or fava beans	¼ cup raw unsalted nuts and/or seeds	1 piece or cup of fresh fruit	4 slices organic dried mango	¼ cup raw unsalted nuts and/or seeds
Dinner	Meatless Monday Stir Fry	Saffron Risotto Crispy Brussels Sprouts	Seitan Picatta with Kale and Quinoa	Tofu Bowl with Charred Scallions Over Vanilla Infused Rice	Flash-Fried Kale Salad with Eggplant and Walnuts Frittata with Broccoli, Tomatoes, and Feta Cheese	Butter Lettuce Salad with Tomatoes, Avocado and Chickpeas Banza Penne with Liguria-Inspired Pesto	Middle Eastern-Inspired Stuffed Eggplant with Tomato and Cucumber Salad
Dessert	Moroccan Orange Salad	Vegan Vanilla Bean Rice Pudding		Vegan Chocolate Mousse	Vegan Chocolate Chip Cookies		Vegan Nice Cream

Vegan Meal Plan 1*

Meal	Monday	Tuesday	Wednesday	Thursday	Friday	Saturday	Sunday
Breakfast	Overnight Oats, Swiss Müesli Style 1 cup berries/fruit on the side	Morning Power Açai Bowl 1 slice Three Seed Bread	Steel-Cut Oatmeal with Cardamom, Cinnamon, Walnuts, and Maple Syrup 1 cup berries/fruit on the side	Morning Antioxidant Smoothie Tofu Scramble	Morning Power Açai Bowl 1 slice Three Seed Bread	Vegan Greek Yogurt Parfait Vegan Thumbprint Corn Muffin	Morning Antioxidant Smoothie Fluffy Whole Wheat Vegan Pancakes with Maple Butter
Lunch	Go-To Lunch Salad with Hearts of Romaine, Cherry Tomatoes, Cucumber, Avocado, Walnuts, and Plant-Based Protein. Roasted Sweet Potato with Sautéed Spinach and Cashew Cream	Classic Lentil Soup Tofurkey, Lettuce, Tomato, Avocado, and Cheese Toast	Summer Salad Chickpea "Caponata" 1 slice Three Seed Bread	Baby Arugula Salad with Roasted Beets, Lentils, and Walnuts Avocado Toast with Tempeh, Tomato, and Mustard Vegenaise	Vegan Macro Bowl	Go-To Lunch Salad with Hearts of Romaine, Cherry Tomatoes, Cucumber, Avocado, Walnuts, and Plant-Based Protein Almond Flour Tortilla Flatbread	Classic Lentil Soup Flash-Fried Kale Salad with Eggplant and Walnuts 1 slice Pan-Fried Sourdough Bread
Snack	1 piece or cup of fresh fruit of your choice	¼ cup raw unsalted nuts and/or seeds	4 pieces unsweetened dried mango	¼ cup raw unsalted nuts and/or seeds	¼ cup dried crispy fava beans or chickpeas	¼ cup raw unsalted nuts and/or seeds	1 piece or cup of fresh fruit of your choice
Dinner	Tempeh Stir Fry, with Spinach, Ginger, Garlic, and Soy Sauce	Middle Eastern-Inspired Stuffed Eggplant with Tomato and Cucumber Salad	No-Cream Cream of Asparagus Soup Fusilli with Creamy Mushroom Sauce	Seitan Piccata with Kale and Quinoa Simple Herb Roasted Carrots	Mixed Green Salad with Sundried Tomatoes, Green Olives, Red Radish, and Pine Nuts, with White Balsamic Vinaigrette. Tofu and Broccoli Curry	No-Pasta Minestrone Soup Lemon Farro Risotto with Asparagus	Tempeh Tacos Crispy Brussels Sprouts
Dessert	Vegan Nice Cream	Vegan Chocolate Mousse	Moroccan Orange Salad		Vegan Chocolate Chip Cookies		Vegan Vanilla Bean Rice Pudding

*In order to meet your nutrient requirements, it's important that you take advantage of the malleability of the recipes. Add nuts and seeds to any breakfast dish or salad. Use fortified products when appropriate. Add legumes and plant-based proteins to the Go-To salads. And, make sure to take your supplements.

Vegan Meal Plan 2*

Meal	Monday	Tuesday	Wednesday	Thursday	Friday	Saturday	Sunday
Breakfast	Morning Power Açai Bowl	Tofu Scramble 1 cup berries/fruit on the side	Whole Grain Almond Butter and Strawberry Jam Toast with Banana, Chia Seeds, and Walnuts 1 cup berries/fruit on the side	Morning Antioxidant Smoothie topped with Homemade Granola 1 slice Three Seed Bread	Vanilla Chia Seed Pudding with Cardamom 1 cup berries/fruit on the side	Morning Antioxidant Smoothie Vegan Thumbprint Corn Muffin	Tofu Scramble 1 cup berries/fruit on the side
Lunch	Go-To Lunch Salad with Hearts of Romaine, Cherry Tomatoes, Cucumber, Avocado, Walnuts, and Plant-Based Protein. 1 slice Three Seed Bread	Light and Silky Vegan Sweet Corn Bisque Avocado Toast with Tempeh, Tomato, and Mustard Vegenaise	Go-To Lunch Salad with Hearts of Romaine, Cherry Tomatoes, Cucumber, Avocado, Walnuts, and Plant-Based Protein. 1 slice Three Seed Bread	Baby Arugula Salad with Roasted Beets, Lentils, and Walnuts Almond Flour Tortilla Flatbread	Tofurkey, Lettuce, Tomato, Avocado, and Cheese Sandwich Light and Silky Vegan Sweet Corn Bisque	Summer Salad Chickpea "Caponata" 1 slice Pan-Fried Sourdough Bread	Vegan Macro Bowl
Snack	1 piece or cup of fresh fruit of your choice	¼ cup raw unsalted nuts and/ or seeds	4 pieces unsweetened dried mango	¼ cup raw unsalted nuts and/ or seeds	¼ cup dried crispy fava beans or chickpeas	¼ cup raw unsalted nuts and/ or seeds	1 piece or cup of fresh fruit of your choice
Dinner	Tofu Bowl with Charred Scallions Over Vanilla-Infused Rice Sautéed Zucchini	Vegetarian Tacos	Vegan Macro Bowl	Flash-Fried Kale Salad with Eggplant and Walnuts Tofu Satay	Baked Stuffed Sweet Potato with Cumin-Infused Black Beans, Melted Vegan Cheddar, and Vegan Greek Yogurt. Crispy Brussels Sprouts	Soba Noodles with Tofu and Vegetables in a Miso Broth	Mixed Green Salad with Sundried Tomatoes, Green Olives, Red Radish, and Pine Nuts, with White Balsamic Vinaigrette Meatless Monday Stir Fry
Dessert	Vegan Nice Cream	Vegan Vanilla Bean Rice Pudding	Moroccan Orange Salad		Vegan Chocolate Chip Cookies	Moroccan Orange Salad	

*In order to meet your nutrient requirements, it's important that you take advantage of the malleability of the recipes. Add nuts and seeds to any breakfast dish or salad. Use fortified products when appropriate. Add legumes and plant-based proteins to the Go-To salads. And, make sure to take your supplements.

Bibliography

Introduction

Psihoyos, Louie. *The Game Changers.* Netflix, 2018.

Fulkerson, Lee. *Forks Over Knives.* Monica Beach Media, 2011.

Clark, Melissa. "The Meat Lover's Guide to Eating Less Meat." *The New York Times,* December 31, 2019. https://www.nytimes.com/2019/12/31/dining /flexitarian-eating-less-meat.html.

Hever, Julieanna. "Plant-Based Diets: A Physician's Guide." *The Permanente Journal* 20, no. 3 (Summer 2016): 15-082. https//doi:.org/10.7812/ TPP/15-082.

Newhart, Beth. "More Young, Liberal Americans Identify as Vegan or Vegetarian Than Any Other Group, Little Change from 2012." *Dairy Reporter,* Last modified September 19, 2018. https://www.dairyreporter.com/ Article/2018/08/14/More-young-liberal-Americans-identify-as-vegan-or-vegetarian-than-any-other-group-little-change-from-2012/?utm_ source=Newsletter_SponsoredSpecial&utm_medium=email&utm_ campaign=Newsletter%2BSponsoredSpecial&c=16HhEPChu5CTi4Iw-p%2BP%2FnX2922m3xPAP.

Neff, Roni A., Danielle Edwards, Anne Palmer, Rebecca Ramsing, Allison Righter, and Julia Wolfson. "Reducing Meat Consumption in the USA: A Nationally Representative Survey of Attitudes and Behaviours." *Public Health Nutrition* 21, no. 10 (March 2018): 1835-1844. doi:10.1017/ S1368980017004190.

Curry, Lynne. "Is the Movement to Eat Less Meat Actually Making a Difference?" *Huffington Post,* Last modified July 31, 2019. https://www.huffpost .com/entry/eat-less-meat-environmental-effect_l_5d39d84fe4b 020cd99501f2d.

Reinhart, RJ. "Snapshot: Few Americans Vegetarian or Vegan." Gallup. August 1, 2018. https://news.gallup.com/poll/238328/snapshot-few-americans-vegetarian-vegan.aspx.

McCarthy, Justin and Scott DeKoster. "Four in 10 Americans Have Eaten Plant-Based Meats." Gallup. January 28, 2020. https://news.gallup.com/poll/282989/four-americans-eaten-plant-based-meats.aspx.

Part One: The Plant-Based Life

What Is a Plant-Based Diet?

Campbell, T. Colin, and Thomas M. Campbell II. *The China Study: The Most Comprehensive Study of Nutrition Ever Conducted and the Startling Implications for Diet, Weight Loss, and Long-Term Health.* Dallas: BenBella Books, 2004.

Stuart, Tristram. *The Bloodless Revolution: A Cultural History of Vegetarianism from 1600 to Modern Times.* London: Harper Press, 2006.

Why Now?

Afshin, Ashkan, Patrick John Sur, Kairsten A. Fay, Leslie Cornaby, Giannina Ferrara, Joseph S. Salama, and Erin C. Mullany, et al. "Health Effects of Dietary Risks in 195 Countries, 1990-2017: A Systematic Analysis for the Global Burden of Disease Study 2017." *The Lancet* 393, no. 10184 (April 2019): 1958-1972. https://doi.org/10.1016/S0140-673(19)30041-8.

Hemler, Elena C., and Frank B. Hu. "Plant-Based Diets for Personal, Population, and Planetary Health." *Advances in Nutrition* 10, no. 4 (November 2019): S275-S283. https://doi.org/10.1093/advances/nmy117.

Centers for Disease Control and Prevention. "Obesity and Overweight." Last modified June 13, 2016. https://www.cdc.gov/nchs/fastats/obesity-overweight.htm.

Hales, Craig M., Margaret D. Carroll, Cheryl D. Fryar, and Cynthia L. Ogden. "Prevalence of Obesity and Severe Obesity Among Adults: United States, 2017-2018." *NCH Data Brief* 360 (February 2020): 1-7. https://www.cdc.gov/nchs/data/databriefs/db360-h.pdf.

World Health Organization. "Cardiovascular Diseases." Last modified May 17, 2017. https://www.who.int/en/news-room/fact-sheets/detail/cardiovascular-diseases-(cvds).

World Health Organization. "Cancer." Last modified September 12, 2018. https://www.who.int/news-room/fact-sheets/detail/cancer.

World Health Organization. "Diabetes." Last modified June 8, 2020. https://www.who.int/news-room/fact-sheets/detail/diabetes.

Garg Shikha, Lindsay Kim, Michael Whitaker, Alissa O'Halloran, Charisse Cummings, Rachel Holstein, Mila Prill, et al. "Hospitalization Rates and Characteristics of Patients Hospitalized with Laboratory-Confirmed Coronavirus Disease 2019-COVID-NET, 14 States, March 1-30, 2020." *MMWR Morb Mortal Wkly Rep* 69, no. 15. (April 17, 2020): 458-464. http://dx.doi.org/10.15585/mmwr.mm6915e3external icon.

Neff, Roni A. Danielle Edwards, Anne Palmer, Rebecca Ramsing, Allison Righter, and Julia Wolfson. "Reducing Meat Consumption in the USA: A Nationally Representative Survey of Attitudes and Behaviors." *Public Health Nutrition* 21, no. 10 (March 2018): 1835-1844. doi:10.1017/S1368980017004190.

Searchinger, Tim, Richard Waite, Craig Hanson, and Janet Ranganathan. "Creating a Sustainable Food Future." *World Resources Report*, December 2018. https://research.wri.org/sites/default/files/2019-07/creating-sustainable-food-future_2_5.pdf.

Womenshealth.gov. "Polycystic Ovary Syndrome." Accessed June 3, 2020. https://www.womenshealth.gov/a-z-topics/polycystic-ovary-syndrome.

Beezhold, Bonnie L., Carol S. Johnston, and Deanna R. Daigle. "Vegetarian diets are associated with healthy mood states: a cross-sectional study in Seventh Day Adventist adults." *Nutr J* 9, no. 26 (June 1, 2010): 1-7. https://doi.org/10.1186/1475-2891-9-26.

Martínez-González, Miguel A., Ana Sánchez-Tainta, Dolores Corella, Jordi Salas-Salvadó, Emilio Ros, Fernando Arós, et al. "A Provegetarian Food Pattern and Reduction in Total Mortality in the Prevención Con Dieta Mediterránea (PREDIMED) Study." *American Journal of Clinical Nutrition* 100, no.1 (December 2014): 320S-328S. https://doi.org/10.3945/ajcn.113.071431.

Safran Foer, Jonathan. "Why We Must Cut out Meat and Dairy before Dinner to Save the Planet." *The Guardian*. September 28, 2019. https://www.theguardian.com/books/2019/sep/28/meat-of-the-matter-the-inconvenient-truth-about-what-we-eat.

Intergovernmental Panel on Climate Change. "Land is a Critical Resource, IPCC Report Says." Accessed June 4, 2020.

https://www.ipcc.ch/2019/08/08/land-is-a-critical-resource_srccl/.

United States Department of Agriculture Economic Research Service - Climate Change. "Climate Change." Accessed April 2, 2020. https://www.ers.usda.gov/topics/natural-resources-environment/climate-change/.

Afshin, Ashkan, Patrick John Sur, Kairsten A. Fay, Leslie Cornaby, Giannina Ferrara, Joseph S. Salama, Erin C. Mullany, et al. "Health Effects of Dietary Risks in 195 Countries, 1990-2017: a systematic analysis for the

Global Burden of Disease Study 2017." *The Lancet* 393, no. 10184 (May 11, 2019): 1958-1972. doi.org/10.3410/f.735450328.793558526.

NASA. "Scientific Consensus: Earth's Climate is Warming." Accessed June 3, 2020. https://climate.nasa.gov/scientific-consensus/.

United Nations. "Climate Change." Accessed June 4, 2020. https://www.un.org/en/sections/issues-depth/climate-change/.

Hemler, Elena C., and Frank B Hu. "Plant-Based Diets for Personal, Population, and Planetary Health." *Advances in Nutrition* 10, no. 4 (November 2019): S275-S283. https://doi.org/10.1093/advances/nmy117.

United States Department of Agriculture Economic Research Service - Climate Change. "Climate Change." Accessed April 2, 2020. https://www.ers.usda.gov/topics/natural-resources-environment/climate-change/.

Climate Nexus. "Animal Agriculture's Impact on Climate Change." Accessed June 4, 2020. https://climatenexus.org/climate-issues/food/animal-agricultures-impact-on-climate-change/.

United States Geological Survey Science for a Changing World. "Watersheds and Drainage Basins." Accessed June 3, 2020.

https://www.usgs.gov/special-topic/water-science-school/science/watersheds-and-drainage-basins?qt-science_center_objects=0#qt-science_center_objects.

Water Footprint Calculator. "Food's Big Water Footprint." April 25, 2020.

https://www.watercalculator.org/footprint/foods-big-water-footprint/.

Springmann, Marco, Keith Wiebe, Daniel Mason-D'Croz, Timothy B. Sulser, Mike Rayner, and Peter Scarborough. "Health and Nutritional Aspects of Sustainable Diet Strategies and Their Association with Environmental Impacts: A Global Modelling Analysis with Country-Level Detail." *Lancet* 2, no. 10 (October 2018): e451–461. https://www.thelancet.com/journals/lanpla/article/PIIS2542-5196(18)30206-7/fulltext.

Humane Society International. "Plant-Based Eating." Accessed June 4, 2020.

https://www.hsi.org/issues/plant-based-eating/.

Foods That Fit...or Don't

Howard, Jacqueline. "Where Do We Stand on Soy?" CNN, March 29, 2018.

https://www.cnn.com/2017/03/07/health/soy-foods-history-cancer-where-do-we-stand-explainer/index.html.

Taylor, Marygrace and Kate Rockwood. "Is Soy Good or Bad for You? Here's the Science-Backed Answer." *Good Housekeeping*, May 17, 2021.

https://www.goodhousekeeping.com/health/diet-nutrition/a20707020/is-soy-good-or-bad-for-you/.

Buettner, Dan. *The Blue Zones*. Washington, D.C.: National Geographic Society, 2008.

Blue Zones. "Why Japan's Longest-Lived Women Hold the Key to Better Health." Last modified April 7, 2015. https://www.bluezones.com/2016/10/japans-longest-lived-women-hold-key-better-health/.

Rizzo, Gianluca and Luciana Baroni. "Soy, Soy Foods and Their Role in Vegetarian Diets." *Nutrients* 10, no. 1 (January 5, 2018): 43. 10.3390/nu10010043.

Jefferson, Wendy N. "Adult Ovarian Function Can Be Affected by High Levels of Soy." *Journal of Nutrition* 140, no. 12 (October 2010): 2322S-2325S. https://doi.org/10.3945/jn.110.123802.

US Soybean Export Council. "Recommended Soy Intakes." Accessed June 4, 2020.

https://ussec.org/wp-content/uploads/2015/10/SOY13_9_Recommended-Soy-Intakes.pdf.

Tsuchiya, Masaki, Tsutomu Miura, Tomoyuki Hanaoka, Motoki Iwasaki, Hiroshi Sasaki, Tadao Tanaka, Hiroyuki Nakao, et al. "Effect of Soy Isoflavones on Endometriosis: Interaction with Estrogen Receptor 2 Gene Polymorphism." *Epidemiology* 18, no. 3 (May 2007): 402-408. doi: 10.1097/01.ede.0000257571.01358.f9.

Messina, Mark, and Geoffrey Redmond. "Effects of Soy Protein and Soybean Isoflavones on Thyroid Function in Healthy Adults and Hypothyroid Patients: A Review of the Literature." *Journal of the American Thyroid Association* 16, no. 3 (March 2006): 249-258. doi: 10.1089/thy.2006.16.249.

Polak, Rani, Edward M. Phillips, and Amy Campbell. "Legumes: Health Benefits and Culinary Approaches to Increase Intake." *Clinical Diabetes* 33, no. 4 (October 2015): 198-205. doi: 10.2337/diaclin.33.4.198.

Harvard T.H. Chan School of Public Health. "Are Anti-Nutrients Harmful?" Accessed June 4, 2020. https://www.hsph.harvard.edu/nutritionsource/anti-nutrients/.

Hu, Frank B., Meir J. Stampfer, Eric B. Rimm, JoAnn E. Manson, Alberto Ascherio, Graham A. Colditz, Bernard A. Rosner, et al. "A Prospective Study of Egg Consumption and Risk of Cardiovascular Disease in Men and Women." *Jama* 281, no. 15 (April 1999): 1387-1394. doi:10.1001/jama.281.15.1387.

United States Department of Health and Human Services and United States Department of Agriculture. *2015-2020 Dietary Guidelines for Americans*. 8th Edition. December 2015. http://health.gov/dietaryguidelines/2015/guidelines/.

Thorning, Tanja Kongerslev, Anne Raben, Tine Tholstrup, Sabita S. Soedamah-Muthu, Ian Givens, and Arne Astrup. "Milk and Dairy Products: Good or Bad for Human Health? An Assessment of the Totality of Scientific Evidence." *Food & Nutrition* 60, no. 32527 (October 2016): http://dx.doi.org/10.3402/fnr.v60.32527.

American Heart Association. "Milk Products." Accessed June 4, 2020. https://www.heart.org/en/healthy-living/healthy-eating/eat-smart/nutrition-basics/dairy-products-milk-yogurt-and-cheese.

Koskinen, Tim T., Heli E.K. Virtanen, Sari Voutilainen, Jaako Mursu, Jyrki K. Virtanen, and Tomi-Pekka Tuomainen. "Intake of Fermented and Non-Fermented Dairy Products and Risk of Incident CHD: the Kuopio Ischaemic Heart Disease Risk Factor Study." *British Journal of Nutrition* 120, no. 11 (December 2018): 1288-01297. https://doi.org/10.1017/S0007114518002830.

National Institute of Health. "Lactose Intolerance." Accessed June 4, 2020. https://ghr.nlm.nih.gov/condition/lactose-intolerance#statistics.

European Society of Cardiology. "Current Advice to Limit Dairy Intake Should be Reconsidered." Last modified August 2018. https://www.escardio.org/The-ESC/Press-Office/Press-releases/Current-advice-to-limit-dairy-intake-should-be-reconsidered.

Juhl, Christian R., Helle K.M. Bergholdt, Iben M. Miller, Gregor B.E. Jemec, Jørgen K. Kanters, and Christian Ellervik. "Dairy Intake and Acne Vulgaris: A Systematic Review and Meta-Analysis of 78,529 Children, Adolescents and Young Adults." *Nutrients* 10, no. 8. (August 2018): 1049-1062. doi:10.3390/nu10081049.

Virtanen Jyrki K., Dariush Mozaffarian, Stephanie E. Chiuve, and Eric B. Rimm. "Fish Consumption and Risk of Major Chronic Disease in Men." *Am J Clin Nutr* 88, no. 6 (December 2008): 1618-1625. doi: 10.3945/ajcn.2007.25816.

Mayo Clinic. "Omega-3 in Fish: How Eating Fish Helps Your Heart." Last modified September 28, 2019. https://www.mayoclinic.org/diseases-conditions/heart-disease/in-depth/omega-3/art-20045614.

Jones, Keithly, Mildred Haley, and Alex Melton. "Per Capita Red Meat and Poultry Disappearance: Insights into Its Steady Growth." *United States Department of Agriculture Economic Research Service*, June 2020. https://www.ers.usda.gov/amber-waves/2018/june/per-capita-red-meat-and-poultry-disappearance-insights-into-its-steady-growth/.

Water Footprint Calculator. "The 900 Gallon Diet: Meat, Portion Size and Water Footprints." Last modified April 2020. https://www.watercalculator.org/footprint/meat-portions-900-gallons/.

Hemler, Elena C., and Frank B. Hu. "Plant-Based Diets for Personal, Population, and Planetary Health." *Advances in Nutrition* 10, no. 4 (November 2019): S275-S283. https://doi.org/10.1093/advances/nmy117.

United States Department of Health and Human Services and United States Department of Agriculture. *Dietary Guidelines for Americans 2015-2020.* 8th Edition. December 2015. http://health.gov/dietaryguidelines/2015/guidelines/.

Not All Plant-Based Diets Are Created Equal

Zong, Geng, Benjamin Lebwohl, Frank B. Hu, Laura Sampson, Lauren W. Dougherty, Walter C. Willett, et al. "Gluten Intake and Risk of Type 2 Diabetes in Three Large Prospective Cohort Studies of US Men and Women." *Diabetologia* 61, no. 10 (October 2018): 2164-2173.

Part Two: The Guide

Verma, Meghna, Raquel Hontecillas, Nuria Tubau-Juni, Vida Abedi, and Josep Bassaganya-Riera. "Challenges in Personalized Nutrition and Health." *Frontiers in Nutrition* 5, no.117 (November 2018): 1–10. https://doi.org/10.3389/fnut.2018.00117.

Springmann, Marco, Keith Wiebe, Daniel Mason-D'Croz, Timothy B. Sulser, Mike Rayner, and Peter Scarborough. "Health and Nutritional Aspects of Sustainable Diet Strategies and Their Association with Environmental Impacts: A Global Modelling Analysis with Country-Level Detail." *Lancet* 2, no. 10 (October 2018): e451–461. https://www.thelancet.com/journals/lanpla/article/PIIS2542-5196(18)30206-7/fulltext.

United States Department of Health and Human Services. *Physical Activity Guidelines for Americans.* 2nd Edition. 2018. https://health.gov/sites/default/files/2019-09/Physical_Activity_Guidelines_2nd_edition.pdf.

Peng, Mei. "How Does Plate Size Affect Estimated Satiation and Intake for Individuals in Normal-Weight and Overweight Groups?" *Obesity Science and Practice* 3, no. 3 (June 2017): 282-288. https://doi.org/10.1002/osp4.119.

Sharp, David, Jeffery Sobal, and Elaine Wethington. "Do Adults Draw Differently-Sized Meals on Larger or Smaller Plates? Examining Plate Size in a Community Sample." *Food Quality and Preference*, 74 (June 2019): 72-77. https://doi.org/10.1016/j.foodqual.2019.01.012.

La Marra, Marco, Giorgio Caviglia, and Raffaella Perrella. "Using Smartphones When Eating Increases Caloric Intake in Young People: An Overview of the Literature." *Frontiers in Psychology*, 11 (December 2020): https://doi.org/10.3389/fpsyg.2020.587886.

Robinson, Eric, Paul Aveyard, Amanda Daley, Kate Jolly, Amanda Lewis, Deborah Lycett, and Suzanne Higgs. "Eating Attentively. A Systematic Review and Meta-Analysis of the Effect of Food Intake Memory and Awareness on Eating." *The American Journal of Clinical Nutrition* 97, no. 4 (April 2013): 728-742. https://doi.org/10.3945/ajcn.112.045245.

Paoli, Antonio, Grant Tinsley, Antonino Bianco, and Tatiana Moro. "The Influence of Meal Frequency and Timing on Health in Humans." *Nutrients* 11, no. 4 (March 2019): 719. https://doi.org/10.3390/nu11040719.

Part Three: The Diets

Diet 1: The Flexitarian

American Dialect Society. "2003 Words of the Year." Accessed August 16, 2020. https://www.americandialect.org/2003_words_of_the_year.

Derbyshire, Emma J. "Flexitarian Diets and Health: A Review of the Evidence-Based Literature." *Frontiers in Nutrition* 3, no. 55 (January 2017): 1–8. https://doi.org/10.3389/fnut.2016.00055.

United States Department of Health and Human Services and United States Department of Agriculture. *Dietary Guidelines for Americans 2015-2020.* 8th Edition. December 2015. http://health.gov/dietaryguidelines/2015/guidelines/.

Halloran, Jean, Meg Bohne, Lena Brook, Sasha Stashwick, Kari Hamerschlag, Cameron Harsh, Steve Roach, and Matt Wellington. "How Top Restaurants Rate on Reducing Use of Antibiotics in Their Meat Supply." Chain Reaction III. September 27, 2017. https://1bps6437gg8c169i-0y1drtgz-wpengine.netdna-ssl.com/wp-content/uploads/2017/09/Chain-Reaction-III.pdf.

Zheng, Wei, and Sang-Ah Lee. "Well-done Meat Intake, Heterocyclic Amine Exposure, and Cancer Risk." *Nutrition Cancer* 61, no. 4 (January 2010): 437–446. https://doi.org10.1080/01635580802710741.

National Cancer Institute. "Chemicals in Meat Cooked at High Temperatures and Cancer Risk." Accessed August 16, 2020. https://www.cancer.gov/about-cancer/causes-prevention/risk/diet/cooked-meats-fact-sheet.

Consumer Reports. "Why Grass-Fed Beef Costs More." Last modified August 24, 2015. https://www.consumerreports.org/cro/magazine/2015/08/why-grass-fed-beef-costs-more/index.htm.

Macronutrient Recommendations: United States Department of Health and Human Services and United States Department of Agriculture. *Dietary Guidelines for Americans 2015-2020*. 8th Edition. December 2015. https://health.gov/our-work/food-nutrition/2015-2020-dietary-guidelines/guidelines/appendix-7/.

Diet 2: The Pescatarian

Johns Hopkins Bloomberg School of Public Health. "School Awarded Scholars' Program Grant from Meatless Monday Campaign." Last modified June 11, 2003. https://www.jhsph.edu/news/news-releases/2003/meatless-scholars.html.

Sifferlin, Alexandra. "Los Angeles City Council Declares Mondays 'Meatless.'" *Time*, November 12, 2012. https://healthland.time.com/2012/11/12/los-angeles-city-council-declares-mondays-meatless/.

Hirsh, Sophie. "Meatless Mondays Expand to All 1,800 New York City Public Schools." Green Matters. Accessed August 16, 2020. https://www.green-matters.com/p/meatless-mondays-nyc-public-schools.

Monterey Bay Seafood Watch. "Seafood Recommendations." Accessed August 16, 2020. https://www.seafoodwatch.org/seafood-recommendations.

Mosher, Lindsay. "What is Sustainable Seafood and How do I Choose It? Your Top Questions Answered." The Oceanic Society. Accessed August 17, 2020. https://www.oceanicsociety.org/blog/2181/what-is-sustainable-seafood-and-how-do-i-choose-it-your-top-questions-answered?gclid=EAIaIQobChMIx_T0wf_J6QIVFo_ICh2zmQpLEAAYASAAEgIeQPD_BwE

ChooseMyPlate, United States Department of Agriculture. "10 Tips: Eat Seafood Twice a Week." Accessed August 16, 2020. https://www.choosemyplate.gov/ten-tips-eat-seafood.

Kantor, Linda. "Americans' Seafood Consumption Below Recommendations." Last modified October 3, 2016. https://www.ers.usda.gov/amber-waves/2016/october/americans-seafood-consumption-below-recommendations/.

Picklo, Matthew. "Eat Fish! Which Fish? That Fish! Go Fish!" Last modified April 2, 2020. https://www.ars.usda.gov/plains-area/gfnd/gfhnrc/docs/news-2013/eat-fish-which-fish-that-fish-go-fish/.

Harvard T.H. Chan School of Public Health. "Fish: Friend or Foe?" Accessed August 16, 2020. https://www.hsph.harvard.edu/nutritionsource/fish/.

Wadyka, Sally. "How Often Should You Be Eating Fish?" Consumer Reports. Last modified May 17, 2018. https://www.consumerreports.org/healthy-eating/how-often-should-you-be-eating-fish/.

University of the Basque Country. "Extra Virgin Olive Oil is the Best Option for Frying Fish." *ScienceDaily*. Accessed August 17, 2020. www.sciencedaily.com/releases/2016/07/160715114736.htm.

United States Environmental Protection Agency. "Should I Be Concerned About Eating Fish and Shellfish?" Accessed August 17, 2020. https://www.epa.gov/choose-fish-and-shellfish-wisely/should-i-be-concerned-about-eating-fish-and-shellfish.

Bes-Rastrollo, M., A. Sánchez-Villegas, C. de la Fuente, J. de Irala, J. A. Martínez, and M. A. Martínez-González. "Olive oil consumption and weight change: the SUN prospective cohort study." *Lipids* 41, no. 3 (March 2006): 249–256. https://doi.org/10.1007/s11745-006-5094-6.

Wyrick, Julianne. "The New/Old Way to Get Your Daily Dose of Olive Oil." *Scientific American*, October 25, 2013. https://blogs.scientificamerican.com/food-matters/the-newold-way-to-get-your-daily-dose-of-olive-oil/.

Diet 3: The Vegetarian

McEvoy, Claire T., Norman Temple, and Jayne V. Woodside. "Vegetarian Diets, Low-Meat Diets and Health: A Review." *Public Health Nutrition* 15, no. 12 (April 2012): 2287–2294. https://doi.org/10.1017/S1368980012000936.

Key, Timothy J., Paul N. Appleby, and Magdalena S. Rosell. "Health Effects of Vegetarian and Vegan Diets." *The American Journal of Clinical Nutrition* 89, no. 5 (March 2009): 1627S–1633S. https://doi.org/10.3945/ajcn.2009.26736N.

Orlich, Michael J., Pramil N. Singh, Joan Sabate, Karen Jaceldo-Siegl, Jing Fan, Synnove Knutsen, W. Lawrence Beeson, and Gary E. Fraser. "Vegetarian Dietary Patterns and Mortality in Adventist Health Study 2." *Jama Internal Medicine* 173, no. 13 (July 2013): 1230–1238. https://doi.org/10.1001/jamainternmed.2013.6473.

Tonstad, Serena, Terry Butler, Ru Yan, and Gary E. Fraser. "Type of Vegetarian Diet, Body Weight, and Prevalence of Type 2 Diabetes." *Diabetes Care* 32, no. 5 (May 2009): 791–796. https://doi.org/10.2337/dc08-1886.

Appleby, Paul N., Margaret Thorogood, Jim I. Mann, and Timothy J.A. Key. "The Oxford Vegetarian Health Study: An Overview." *American Journal of Clinical Nutrition* 70 (1999): 525S–31S.

McEvoy, Claire T. "Vegetarian Diets, Low-Meat Diets and Health: A Review." *Public Health Nutrition* 15, no. 12 (April 2012): 2287–2294. https://doi. org/10.1017/S1368980012000936.

Rizzo, Nico S., Karen Jaceldo-Siegl, Joan Sabate, and Gary E. Fraser. "Nutrient Profiles of Vegetarian and Nonvegetarian Dietary Patterns." *J Acad Nutr Diet* 113, no. 12 (December 2013): 1610–1619. https://www.ncbi.nlm.nih. gov/pmc/articles/PMC4081456/.

Davey, Gwyneth K., Elizabeth A. Spencer, Paul N. Appleby, Naomi E. Allen, Katherine H. Knox, and Timothy J. Key. "EPIC-Oxford: Lifestyle Charac- teristics and Nutrient Intakes in a Cohort of 33 883 Meat-Eaters and 31 546 Non-Meat Eaters in the UK." *Public Health Nutrition* 6, no. 3 (June 2002): 259–268. https://doi.org/10.1079/PHN2002430.

Key, Timothy J.A., Gwyneth K. Davey, and Paul N. Appleby. "Health Bene- fits of a Diet." *Proceedings of the Nutrition Society* 58 (1999): 271–275. https://www.cambridge.org/core/services/aop-cambridge-core/content /view/8774207AE8B2CCB4A90D6ADDBC9EA89F/S00296651 99000373a.pdf/health_benefits_of_a_vegetarian_diet.pdf.

Baboumian, Patrik. "What About Protein?" Accessed August 18, 2020, https:// gamechangersmovie.com/food/protein/.

Centers for Disease Control and Prevention. "Only 1 in 10 Adults Get Enough Fruits or Vegetables." Last modified November 16, 2017. https://www.cdc. gov/media/releases/2017/p1116-fruit-vegetable-consumption.html.

Mangels, Ann Reed. "Bone Nutrients for Vegetarians." *The American Journal of Clinical Nutrition* 100, no. 1 (July 2014): 469S–475S. https://doi. org/10.3945/ajcn.113.071423.

Pawlak, Roman, Julia Berger, and Ian Hines. "Iron Status of Vegetarian Adults: A Review of Literature." *American Journal of Lifestyle Medicine* 12, no. 6 (November 2018): 486–498. https://doi.org/10.1177/1559827616682933.

National Institutes of Health. "Iron Fact Sheet for Health Professionals." Last modified February 28, 2020. https://ods.od.nih.gov/factsheets/Iron -HealthProfessional/.

Diet 4: The Vegan

Richter, Margrit, Heiner Boeing, Dorle Grünewald-Funk, Helmut Heseker, Anja Kroke, Eva Leschik-Bonnet, Helmut Oberritter, Daniela Strohm, and Bernhard Watzl. "Vegan Diet: Position for the German Nutrition Society (DGE)." *Ernaehrungs Umschau* 63, no. 4 (April 2016): 92–102.https://doi. org/10.4455/eu.2016.021.

Glick-Bauer, Marian and Ming-Chin Yeh. "The Health Advantage of a Vegan Diet: Exploring the Gut Microbiota Connection." *Nutrients* 6, no. 11 (2014): 4822–4838. https://doi.org/10.3390/nu6114822.

Heiner Boeing, Dorle Grünewald-Funk, Helmut Heseker, Anja Kroke, Eva Leschik-Bonnet, Helmut Oberritter, Daniela Strohm, and Bernhard Watzl. "Vegan Diet: Position for the German Nutrition Society (DGE)." *Ernaehrungs Umschau* 63, no. 4 (April 2016): 92–102. https://: doi.org/10.4455/eu.2016.021.

Leitzmann, Claus. "Vegetarian Nutrition: Past, Present, Future." *The American Journal of Clinical Nutrition* 100, no. 1 (July 2014): 496S–592S. https://doi.org/10.3945/ajcn.113.071365.

Branch, Jessica. "Boost Nutrition and Flavor with these Tips." Consumer Reports. Last modified September 27, 2019. https://www.consumer-reports.org/fruits-vegetables/vegetables-that-are-healthier-cooked/.

Pawlak, R., S.E. Lester, and T. Babatunde. "The Prevalence of Cobalamin Deficiency Among Vegetarians Assessed By Serum Vitamin B-12: A Review of Literature." *European Journal of Clinical Nutrition* 68 (March 2014): 541–548. https://doi.org/10.1038/ejcn.2014.46.

National Institute of Health. "Omega-3 Fatty Acids: Fact Sheet For Health Professionals." Last modified October 17, 2019. https://ods.od.nih.gov/factsheets/Omega3FattyAcids-HealthProfessional/#h2.

American Pregnancy Association. "Omega-3 Fatty Acids: FAQs." Last modified April 25, 2013. https://americanpregnancy.org/health-fitness/omega-3-fatty-acids-faqs-4922.

Greenberg, James, Stacey J. Bell, and Wendy Van Ausdal. "Omega-3 Fatty Acid Supplementation During Pregnancy." *Reviews in Obstetrics and Gynecology* 1, no. 4 (2008): 162–169. https://www.ncbi.nlm.nih.gov/pmc/articles/PMC2621042/.

Part Four: The Recipes

Buettner, Dan. "Blue Zones Diet: Food Secrets of the World's Longest-Lived People." *Blue Zones*, July 5, 2021. https://www.bluezones.com/2020/07/blue-zones-diet-food-secrets-of-the-worlds-longest-lived-people/.

Brookie, Kate L., Georgia I. Best, and Tamlin S. Conner. "Intake of Raw Fruits and Vegetables Is Associated with Better Mental Health Than Intake of Processed Fruits and Vegetables." *Frontiers in Psychology* 9, 487 (2018). doi.org/10.3389/fpsyg.2018.00487.

Acknowledgements

I started writing *The Win-Win Diet* a few months before COVID-19 emerged and finished in January 2021. Despite the incredible trials of that first pandemic year, colleagues, dear friends, and family stood by me as I wrote this book. I could not have done it alone.

I am grateful for the encouragement, patience, kindness, and expertise of my editor, Caitlin Leffel, who was invaluable to my efforts from development through completion of the manuscript. I am thankful to Jeff Wald for introducing me to Anthony Ziccardi and his team at Post Hill Press including Maddie Sturgeon, Megan Wheeler, and Devon Brown, who took a chance on me with their belief that this book should see the light of day. To Abbe Baker for her early copy edits. To Dana Cowin for her invaluable coaching, deep knowledge of food, editorial insight, and always being available in a pinch.

I cannot express enough thanks to all my close friends for tirelessly providing wise counsel. To Heather Hansen for her countless tips on how to advocate for myself and the book. To Elizabeth Ross, Yasmine Nainzedeh, and Elias Guerra, for their devoted friendship, steadfast interest in this project, faith in me, and insistence that I make it to the finish line. To Nancy Reyes McGlaughlin for being my bravest recipe tester. To Bruce Wilcox for reviewing an early draft of the book without judgement. To Amanda Fortini for over two decades of friendship and conversation about writing and nutrition. To Jillian Turecki for helping me clarify the pivot I sought to make in my life before setting out to write this book and instilling me with the confidence to execute it. Thank you to Philip Chong and Caroline Waxler for their marketing savvy and desire to see me go forth unabated in promoting the book. To Juliette Haas for her youthful energy and social media skills. To David and Sandra Haas for sending their daughter my way and always being up for endless discussions about the world of wellness. I am also deeply appreciative to Samhita Jayanti and the talent she sent me in Diana Vives and George Christaras, who could not have been more dedicated to refining my brand and building my new website.

To Diana and Mishal Adam Weston, another incredible team that did a beautiful job on designing my cover in the eleventh hour.

I have enormous gratitude for the mentorship of Dr. Jana Klauer and Dr. Johnathan Tobin. I would never have gone back to school later in life for my Master of Science in Nutrition and Dietetics had it not been for Dr. Klauer's precedent. I could not have been luckier than to have had the incredible opportunity to work with Dr. Tobin on a Rockefeller University nutrition study in collaboration with Dr. Jan Breslow, Dr. Peter Holt, and the rest of their research team. Thank you to Marnie Imhoff and Andrea Ronning for taking an interest in me throughout the duration of that study and beyond.

Many thanks to my New York University professors, Dr. Kristie Lancaster and Dr. Charles Mueller, for championing rigorous scientific research, analysis, and reporting. Your tutelage was fundamental to this effort.

I am appreciative to my entire launch team who helped promote this book on social media, including Dr. Miriam Knoll, Dr. Jaqueline Segelnick, Cassandra Ferland, Jenny Campbell, Deborah Lippmann, Micky Hoogendijk, and everyone else who will be helping down the road. I cannot tell you how valuable every mention is for book sales. To Emi Battaglia for her expertise in public relations and the team at Mouth Digital for their additional support.

And of course, I cannot express enough appreciation for the love and support of my family including Kenneth Lipper, Evelyn Gruss Lipper, Mia Wilcox, Tamara Smith, Daniella Coules, and Joanna Lipper who offered infinite personal support and helpful suggestions along the way.

About the Author

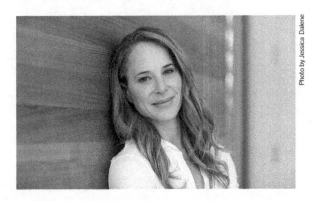

Photo by Jessica Dalene

Julie Wilcox is a wellness consultant, writer, teacher, and coach. She has spent her life exploring how to hone the body, mind, and spirit to become healthier, happier, balanced, and more productive. She believes in personalized solutions that speak to individual needs. We are all unique and deserve specialized attention.

As founder of Julie Wilcox Wellness and co-founder of ISHTA Yoga, Julie has taught thousands of clients individually and through corporate wellness programs. She has piloted ongoing programs with IBM, TBWA\Chiat Day, Marti Hotels & Marinas Group, and Deborah Lippmann Enterprises, among others. Her personal and professional experience are backed by a Master of Science degree in Nutrition and Dietetics from NYU and national certifications in yoga and fitness through the Yoga Alliance of America and ACE™. Julie earned her A.B. at Harvard College.

Julie is continuously engaged, up-to-date, and active at the forefront of her profession. In addition to academic projects taken on as a qualitative researcher and writer (Rockefeller University four-year study on Overweight and Adolescent Obesity Prevention and Management), she is also a content creator whose articles and videos have been featured in *Forbes*, Fox News, MindBodyGreen, *Parade*, Refinery29, and Greatist, to name a few. Her non-profit work is equally wellness-focused. She is a consultant and advisory board member for Quincy Asian Resources (QARI), an NGO providing food security and health and wellness services to underserved immigrant populations, and executive wellness director of Jewish Orthodox Women's Medical Association (JOWMA).